Genital Dermatoses

Genital Dermatoses

Editor-in-Chief

Jayakar Thomas MD DD MNAMS PhD FRCP (Edin, Glasg, Lond, Irel)
FRCPCH FAAD FIAD FIAP

Professor and Head
Department of Dermatology
Sree Balaji Medical College and Hospital, Bharath University
Chennai, Tamil Nadu, India

Editors

Parimalam Kumar MD DD DNB FRCP FIAD

Professor and Head
Department of Dermatology
Government Villupuram Medical College
Villupuram, Tamil Nadu, India

Sindhu Ragavi Balaji MBBS MD

Consultant Dermatologist
Carves Skin Clinic
Chennai, Tamil Nadu, India

Dinesh Kumar Devaraj MBBS MD

Medical Director and Consultant Dermatologist
Vee Care DermatoPlastic
Chennai, Tamil Nadu, India

Foreword

B Parveen

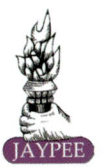

The Health Sciences Publisher
New Delhi | London | Philadelphia | Panama

Jaypee Brothers Medical Publishers (P) Ltd

Headquarters
Jaypee Brothers Medical Publishers (P) Ltd
4838/24, Ansari Road, Daryaganj
New Delhi 110 002, India
Phone: +91-11-43574357
Fax: +91-11-43574314
Email: jaypee@jaypeebrothers.com

Overseas Offices

J.P. Medical Ltd
83 Victoria Street, London
SW1H 0HW (UK)
Phone: +44 20 3170 8910
Fax: +44 (0)20 3008 6180
Email: info@jpmedpub.com

Jaypee-Highlights Medical Publishers Inc
City of Knowledge, Bld. 237, Clayton
Panama City, Panama
Phone: +1 507-301-0496
Fax: +1 507-301-0499
Email: cservice@jphmedical.com

Jaypee Medical Inc
325 Chestnul Street
Suite 412, Philadelphia, PA 19106, USA
Phone: +1 267-519-9789
Email: support@jpmedus.com

Jaypee Brothers Medical Publishers (P) Ltd
17/1-B Babar Road, Block-B, Shaymali
Mohammadpur, Dhaka-1207
Bangladesh
Mobile: +08801912003485
Email: jaypeedhaka@gmail.com

Jaypee Brothers Medical Publishers (P) Ltd
Bhotahity, Kathmandu, Nepal
Phone: +977-9741283608
Email: kathmandu@jaypeebrothers.com

Website: www.jaypeebrothers.com
Website: www.jaypeedigital.com

© 2016, Jaypee Brothers Medical Publishers

The views and opinions expressed in this book are solely those of the original contributor(s)/author(s) and do not necessarily represent those of editor(s) of the book.

All rights reserved. No part of this publication may be reproduced, stored or transmitted in any form or by any means, electronic, mechanical, photocopying, recording or otherwise, without the prior permission in writing of the publishers.

All brand names and product names used in this book are trade names, service marks, trademarks or registered trademarks of their respective owners. The publisher is not associated with any product or vendor mentioned in this book.

Medical knowledge and practice change constantly. This book is designed to provide accurate, authoritative information about the subject matter in question. However, readers are advised to check the most current information available on procedures included and check information from the manufacturer of each product to be administered, to verify the recommended dose, formula, method and duration of administration, adverse effects and contraindications. It is the responsibility of the practitioner to take all appropriate safety precautions. Neither the publisher nor the author(s)/editor(s) assume any liability for any injury and/or damage to persons or property arising from or related to use of material in this book.

This book is sold on the understanding that the publisher is not engaged in providing professional medical services. If such advice or services are required, the services of a competent medical professional should be sought.

Every effort has been made where necessary to contact holders of copyright to obtain permission to reproduce copyright material. If any have been inadvertently overlooked, the publisher will be pleased to make the necessary arrangements at the first opportunity.

Inquiries for bulk sales may be solicited at: jaypee@jaypeebrothers.com

Genital Dermatoses

First Edition: **2016**

ISBN: 978-93-5250-012-3

Printed at Sanat Printers

Dedicated to

Many devoted practitioners who provide skin health to patients with genital dermatoses, our committed teachers of dermatology, the thousands who suffer from genital disorders, and most of all to our spouses for their care, love, and affection without which this humble piece of work would not have been a reality.

Foreword

It is a privilege and pleasure to pen these lines of foreword for a book edited by Professor Jayakar Thomas. I say this because I know him as a voracious reader, popular teacher, and a masterly orator and also a great descriptive writer. I have been reading his several works—original articles, chapters in books, and also his other books.

This book on *genital dermatoses* is one that caters to all levels of medical persons—undergraduate and postgraduate medical students, practicing physicians and consultants in general, and to all dermatologists in particular.

It has been written in a user-friendly style with several color images that are not easy to acquire in Indian patients. Genital Dermatoses is a rational mix of clinical, pathological, and treatment details on this group of dermatologic conditions.

All the contributors deserve to share this honor of compiling this book by putting in immense efforts to publish this book.

It is my opinion that this book needs to be placed in the libraries of all medical institutions and in the hands of all physicians.

I convey to Professor Jayakar Thomas and the other editors all my best wishes to publish more and more informative books in the future.

B Parveen MB DD MD
Former Professor and Head
Department of Dermatology
Madras Medical College
Chennai, Tamil Nadu, India

Preface

"Knowledge, if not shared is of no use at all."

Advances in dermatologic science have been spectacular and we are pleased to present this title *Genital Dermatoses*.

Genital dermatoses is an elusive, complex, and difficult group of diseases to diagnose and treat. Conventional treatments, such as antibiotics, steroids, and antihistamines have proven to be useful for treating a handful of genital dermatoses; they are usually not always effective.

In this book, a wide variety of diagnostic tests and treatments are described, all of which have effectively helped many patients live long, productive lives. We have shared the goal to formulate protocols that treat the underlying cause of disease, rather than just its symptoms.

This title offers a thoroughly updated presentation of the classic pathophysiology, basics of clinical presentation, and the details of the cutting-edge methods and tools that are now available for the assessment of symptoms and the effective management of genital dermatoses. The text is supported by to-the-point photographs, radiographs, illustrations and patient-care algorithms and tables.

We wish all readers a happy and fruitful reading.

Jayakar Thomas
Parimalam Kumar
Sindhu Ragavi Balaji
Dinesh Kumar Devaraj

Contents

CHAPTER 1:	Introduction	1
CHAPTER 2:	Anatomy	2
CHAPTER 3:	History Taking	5
CHAPTER 4:	Clinical Examination	6
CHAPTER 5:	Normal Anatomical Variants	8
CHAPTER 6:	Sexually Transmitted Infections Affecting the Genitalia	10
CHAPTER 7:	Genital Infections Other Than Sexually Transmitted Diseases	97
CHAPTER 8:	Bullous Dermatoses	116
CHAPTER 9:	Inflammatory Lesions of the Genitalia	131
CHAPTER 10:	Premalignant Lesions of the Genitalia	186
CHAPTER 11:	Malignant Conditions	192
CHAPTER 12:	Other Diseases of the Genitalia	198
CHAPTER 13:	Genital Pain Syndrome	214
	Bibliography	219
	Index	223

CHAPTER 1

Introduction

The skin in the genital area is an extension of the skin elsewhere in the body and can be affected by common skin disorders that can affect other areas along with genital area incidentally or can present in the genital areas with unusual features. It can also be affected by conditions that are completely or predominantly confined to this area. As a sexual organ, these areas can also harbor many sexually transmitted infections (STIs).

Most of the disorders affecting the vulva and penis are dermatological, modified by anatomical, hormonal, and microbiological influences. They more often have multifactorial etiology than dermatoses affecting other areas of the body. There is a peculiar challenge in the management of these disorders because majority of the problems are dermatological and the specialists predominantly treating it are gynecologists, urologists, genitourinary physicians, who would have had little or no training in dermatology.

CHAPTER 2

Anatomy

MALE GENITALIA

The male groin area comprises of the penis, scrotum (male genitalia), along with the pubic area, genitocrural folds, perineum, and anus. The penis is the sexual organ and start from the pubic wall and the shaft of the penis toward the distal part is called the glans penis. The groove between the glans and the shaft of the penis is known as the coronal sulcus. The retractable skin (foreskin) covering the glans is also known as the prepuce and the urethra opens as the external urethral meatus at the distal-most point of the penis. The ventral surface of the penis is in contact with scrotum (Fig. 1).

FEMALE GENITALIA

The female external genitalia are collectively referred to as the vulva. It comprises the region known as the urogenital triangle, bounded anteriorly by the symphysis pubis, the pubic rami laterally, and the transverse perineal body posteriorly. The mons pubis, paired labia majora and labia minora, clitoris, and vulval vestibule are present within this area. The mons pubis is softly rounded and is densely covered in hair (Fig. 2).

Anatomy

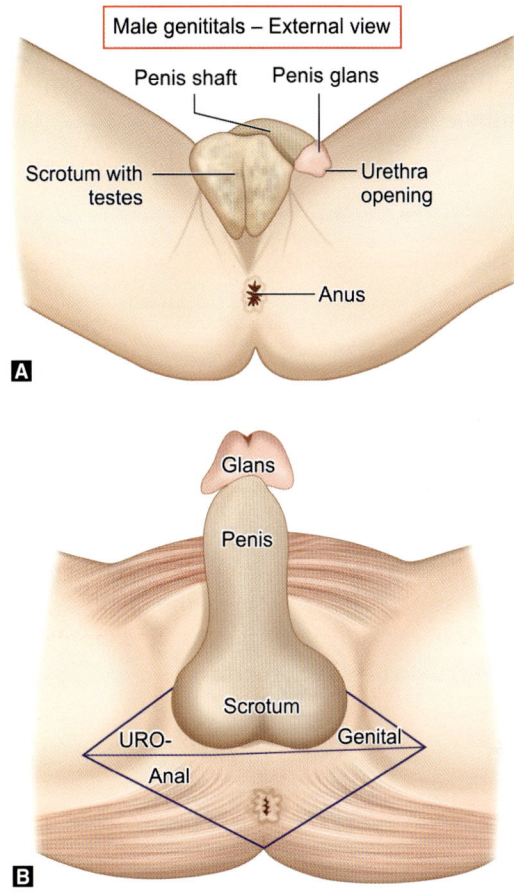

Figure 1: Anatomy of male genitalia.

The labia majora homologue of the scrotum are paired, rounded folds of skin extending downward and backward from the mons pubis, and meet posteriorly in the midline to form the posterior commissure, which lies approximately 2 cm anterior to the anus. The inner aspects of the labia majora fuse into the outer aspects of the labia minora. The interlabial sulci and the labia minora lack hair but the sebaceous glands are prominent. The pudendal cleft contains the vestibule with the openings of the vagina and urethra. Minor (paraurethral) and major (Bartholin's) vestibular glands also open into the vestibule.

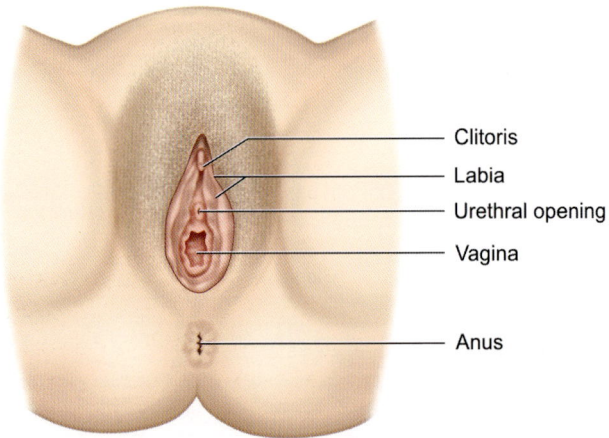

Figure 2: Anatomy of female genitalia

CHAPTER 3

History Taking

Along with the presenting complaint, also ask for burning micturition, uretheral discharge, anogenital itching, skin eruptions, etc. The age of the patient is important as sexually transmitted infections (STIs) would be more common in the younger age group and malignancy would be more common in the older age group. History of any coexisting skin disorders should be sought for, along with sexual contact, behavior history, and medication usage. In a female patient, association with premenstrual exacerbation has to be sought. The female patient also needs to be asked on dyspareunia, treatments that have been used and whether these led to improvement or worsening of symptoms. History of antibiotic usage, and hormonal contraception must be asked for a personal or family history of skin disorders, as is diabetes, autoimmunity, and malignancy.

CHAPTER 4

Clinical Examination

A general skin examination including the nongenital mucosa, hair-bearing areas, flexures, nails, and scalp has to be performed before proceeding to the local examination.

MALE

The external genitalia need to be examined with care for any skin lesions, erosions, eruptions, infestations, etc. The prepuce has to be checked to rule out phimosis and also to examine the coronal sulcus, glans penis, and external urethral meatus closely. The perineum and anus also needs to be examined. The area also needs to be examined with a magnifying lens to make sure the examination is complete. Any samples for investigations like swabs, slides, scrapings or a skin biopsy at times may be required.

FEMALE

The vulval and perianal skin needs to be examined along with as the inguinal and gluteal folds. Features like lichenification, pigmentation, erosions, ulcers, associated vaginitis need to be looked for. The perineum and anus also needs to be examined. The area also needs to be examined with a magnifying lens to make sure the examination is complete. A low vaginal swab has to be

Clinical Examination

taken for microscopy and culture. Biopsy of vulval skin or mucosa can be more distressing and painful to the patient, but may assist in diagnosis. The skin disorders of the genitalia can be grouped into the following categories:
- Normal anatomical variants
- Sexually transmitted infections (STI) affecting the genitals
- Genital infections other than sexually transmitted diseases (STDs)
- Bullous dermatoses
- Inflammatory conditions
- Premalignant dermatoses
- Malignant diseases of genitalia
- Genital pain syndromes.

CHAPTER 5

Normal Anatomical Variants

MALE

Adolescent males usually are concerned about the changes happening in the external genitalia like prominence of hair, sebaceous glands, and veins. Ectopic sebaceous glands, also known as Fordyce spots, can also be a presenting complaint over the scrotal skin and also over the penile shaft. Pearly penile papules are common cause of anxiety among adolescents and can be mistaken for verruca. They are flesh-colored, smooth, rounded, and flat papules around 1–3 mm in size, which occur predominantly over the coronal sulcus. Reassurance and education is what is needed in such situations.

Angiokeratomas are reddish-blue papules occurring over penile shaft or scrotum. These lesions are more common among the whites. Laser or electrocautery ablation can be done, but recurrence is common.

FEMALE

Vestibular papillae are considered a variant of normal and are the female equivalent of penile pearly papules. Vestibular papillae are asymptomatic and, soft micropapules that may be rounded or filiform, located in the vestibule. The papillae are most prominently seen in the posterior aspect and are distributed symmetrically with each papilla arising from its own solitary base. The patient needs to be reassured.

Sebaceous gland hyperplasia on the labia minora are usually numerous and prominent, and are seen as yellow micropapules. Treatment is not necessary.

Varicosities of the labial veins may occur unilaterally in association with limb varicosities, or can appear in pregnancy.

Angiokeratomas are normally asymptomatic, and are found on the labia majora. They can become quite large and bleed, if traumatized, particularly in pregnancy. In pregnancy, the vulva can become hyperpigmented and sometimes varicosities can also develop.

CHAPTER

6

Sexually Transmitted Infections Affecting the Genitalia

Infections affecting the genital skin that are sexually transmitted are caused by bacteria, virus, fungi, and treponemes. Parasitic infestations caused by itch mite and louse can also be sexually transmitted. This section will deal with the sexually transmitted infections (STIs), syndromic approach, and procedure of collection of specimen for examination to confirm diagnosis.

MOLLUSCUM CONTAGIOSUM

Molluscum contagiosum (MC) is a viral infection of the skin or occasionally of the mucous membranes, caused by a DNA poxvirus called the molluscum contagiosum virus (MCV). There are four types of MCV: MCV-1 to -4; MCV-1 is the most prevalent and MCV-2 is seen usually in adults. As with other poxviruses, MC is spread through fomite or skin-to-skin contact, and microscopic abrasions in the epidermis are thought to facilitate transmission. MC infection occurs frequently among children and also affects sexually-active adults, where it is classified among the sexually transmitted diseases (STDs). This common viral disease has a higher incidence in children, sexually active adults, and those who are immunodeficient. The typical MC lesion is an asymptomatic, firm, smooth, round papule with central umbilication. They commonly appear on the suprapubic area when sexually transmitted, although they may affect the penis and inguinal folds (Figs 1 to 3). While most lesions are asymptomatic, they can become painful, if irritated, and can appear very erythematous. Small lesions are easily missed. Differential diagnosis includes genital warts and folliculitis.

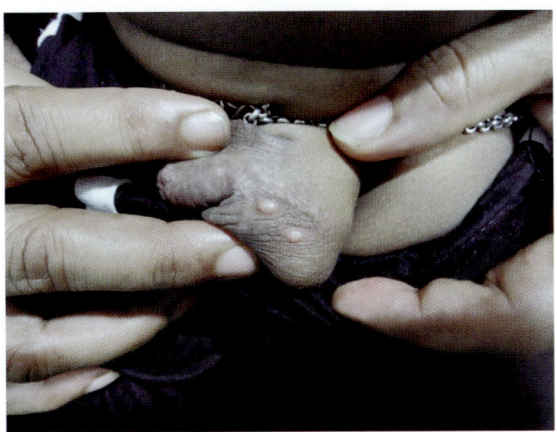

Figure 1: Smooth firm papule with central umbilication seen over scrotum

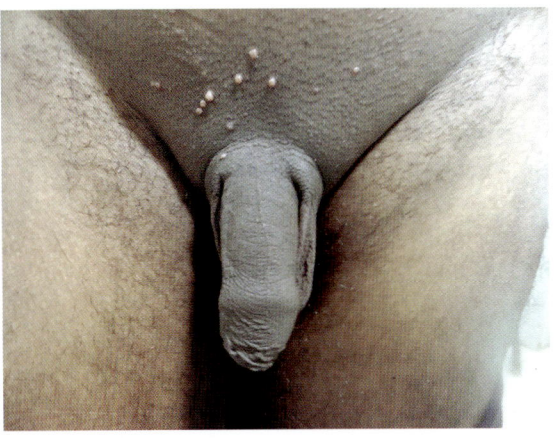

Figure 2: Multiple molluscum contagiosum in a boy

Genital Dermatoses

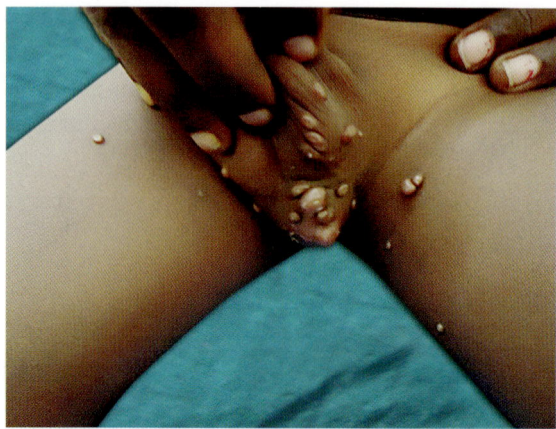

Figure 3: Multiple molluscum contagiosum in a child—child abuse should be ruled out

Diagnosis

The characteristic histologic feature is the presence of large, eosinophilic, intracytoplasmic Henderson-Patterson inclusion bodies. These Henderson-Patterson bodies consist of a membrane sac that contains numerous viral particles. In addition, the histology typically shows epidermal hyperplasia, increased size of basophils, and deep purple basal keratinocytes.

Treatment

Spontaneous disappearance of MC lesions with no residual scarring is common, often after a period of inflammation. Lesion eradication may be mechanical (curettage, laser, or cryotherapy with liquid nitrogen), chemical (trichloroacetic acid, tretinoin), or immunologic (imiquimod).

PEDICULOSIS PUBIS

It is caused by the crab louse *Phthirus pubis*, transmitted by close body contact and may infest the strong hairs of the pubic and perianal areas; those of the legs, forearms, chest, and rarely the eyelashes, eyebrows, axillary hair, and beard. They are spread from person to person usually through sexual contact. They appear as 1-2 mm tan-brown attachments to the hair shaft. Observing movement under magnification can confirm the diagnosis. A central dark area in the louse is noted after feeding. They attach with claws to pubic areas and periodically feed. Several weeks after infestations, patients develop itching. Lice can survive off the human body for up to 24 hours. Nits or eggs may be attached to the hair, typically as 1 mm solid concretions barely visible to the naked eye. They are more easily seen with magnification. Blue spots or macula cerulea may appear on the groin which represent bites. Typically, patients present with complaints of genital itching in the absence of visible lesions. Diagnosis is usually based on typical clinical findings. Microscopic examination of a nit or louse of *P. pubis* may be undertaken, if there is diagnostic uncertainty.

Management

Patients should be advised to avoid close contact until they and their sexual partners have completed treatment and follow-up. All hairy areas of the body from the neck down should be treated.
- Malathion 0.5% lotion on dry hair, wash out 12 hours after application
- Permethrin 1% lotion on wet hair, wash out after 10 minutes.

Treatment may be repeated after 1 week, if necessary. The nits can be removed with a fine-toothed comb.

Sexual partners within the previous month should be treated, preferably simultaneously with the index patient. Sexual contact should be avoided for 1 week following treatment of both partners.

SCABIES

Scabies is a common parasitic infection caused by the mite *Sarcoptes scabiei* variety *hominis,* an arthropod of the order acarina. The mite is an obligate parasite that completes its entire life cycle on humans. Only female mites burrow into the skin. The maturation process

Genital Dermatoses

lasts about 15 days; with the larvae emerging 2-3 days after the eggs are laid. About 5-15 female mites live on a host infected with classic scabies, but the number can reach hundreds or even millions in cases of crusted scabies. The skin eruption of classic scabies is considered a consequence of both infestation and a hypersensitivity reaction to the mite. The incubation period before symptoms appear is 36 weeks for primary infestation, but may be as short as 1-3 days in cases of reinfestation.

The predominant route of transmission is direct skin-to-skin contact. Transmission by means of shared clothing or other indirect method is rare with classic scabies, but may occur with crusted scabies (e.g., in immunocompromised hosts). Sexual transmission also occurs.

Clinical Features

Classic manifestations of scabies include generalized and intense itching, usually sparing the face and head. Pruritus is worst at night. The lesions are located mostly in the finger, on the flexor surfaces of the wrists, on the elbows, in the axillae, on the buttocks, and genitalia. Inflammatory pruritic papules are present at most sites. Burrows and nodules (generally in the genital regions and axillae) are specific for scabies but may be absent. Patients with scabies may develop indurated nodules on the scrotum (Figs 4 and 5). Biopsy will show hypersensitivity reaction presumably to remnants of the scabies mite. The lesion is not infectious. They will resolve over several months or can be treated with intralesional steroids. Nonspecific secondary lesions, including excoriations, eczematization, and impetiginization may occur anywhere. Immunosuppressed patients, such as those with advanced human immunodeficiency virus (HIV) infection may develop what is known as Norwegian scabies, characterized by limited or diffuse hyperkeratotic somewhat yellow plaques, which are literally teeming with million of mites. The degree of immunosuppression accounts for the mite proliferation and absence of itching.

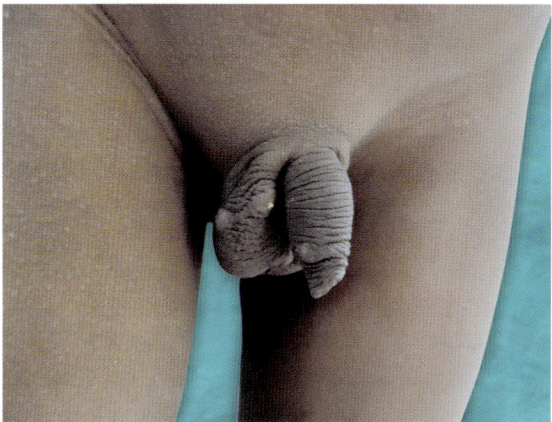

Figure 4: Papules and nodules over scrotum, groin, and shaft of penis in scabies.

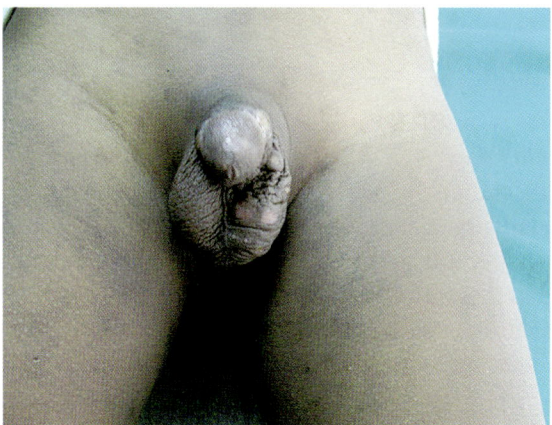

Figure 5: Scabies with secondary infection.

Diagnosis

Definitive diagnosis relies on the identification of mites, eggs, eggshell fragments, or mite pellets. Multiple superficial skin samples should be obtained from characteristic lesions, specifically burrows or papules and vesicles in the site of burrows.

Treatment

Infested persons and their close physical contacts should be treated at the same time regardless of, whether symptoms are present. Permethrin and lindane are the two most studied topical treatments for scabies. 5% permethrin is recommended by the Centers for Disease Control and Prevention (CDC) as first-line topical therapy for scabies. Other topical treatments include benzyl benzoate and crotamiton. Topical treatments may be poorly tolerated by some patients. An alternative approach is the use of oral ivermectin, an agent that has been used extensively for several parasitic infections, including onchocerciasis, lymphatic filariasis, and other nematode-related infestations. Ivermectin is thought to interrupt glutamate-induced and γ-aminobutyric acid-induced neurotransmission in parasites, leading to their paralysis and death. In humans, ivermectin does not cross the intact blood-brain barrier.

CHANCROID

Chancroid is a STD caused by the gram-negative bacterium *Haemophilus ducreyi (H. ducreyi)* and is characterized by necrotizing genital ulceration which may be accompanied by inguinal lymphadenitis or bubo formation. Chancroid may also be spread to other anatomical sites by autoinoculation, a clinical feature first demonstrated experimentally by Ducreyi in 1889. Genital ulceration has been shown to be a major cofactor in the transmission of human immunodeficiency virus type 1 (HIV-1) infection.

Clinical Features

Haemophilus ducreyi initiates an infective process within the genital skin after the formation of epidermal microabrasions during sexual intercourse. A tender, erythematous papule may develop 4–7 days later before progressing to the pustular stage. Pustules often rupture after a further 2–3 days to form painful shallow ulcers with granulomatous bases and purulent exudates. The ulcer edge is typically ragged and undermined (Fig. 6). Lesions typically occur

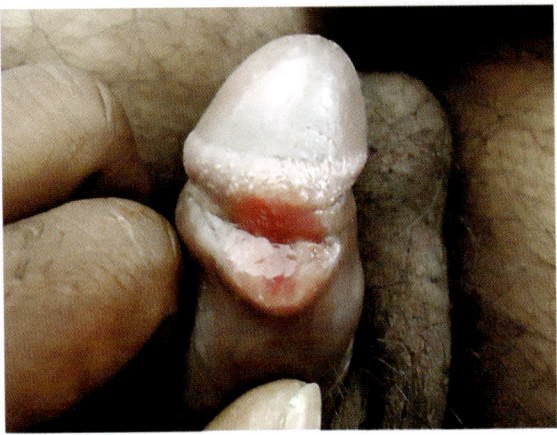

Figure 6: Shallow painful ulcer with granulomatous base in chancroid

on the prepuce and frenulum in men and on the vulva, cervix, and perianal area in women. Complications include phimosis in men and further phagedenic ulceration due to secondary bacterial infection. Extragenital cases of chancroid with lesions on inner thighs, breasts, and fingers have been reported but are rarely seen in clinical practice. Painful, tender inguinal lymphadenitis typically occurs in up to 50% of cases and the lymph nodes may develop into buboes. The lymphadenopathy is usually unilateral and tends to be more prevalent in men. If not aspirated or drained through incision, fluctuant buboes can rupture spontaneously. HIV-seropositive patients have increased number of genital ulcers which may heal at slower rate.

Diagnosis

Chancroid can be diagnosed by employing following methods:
- Culture of material obtained from the ulcer base, or the undermined edges of the ulcer, after removing superficial pus with a cotton-tipped swab, or from pus aspirated from the bubo. The material can be plated directly onto culture medium

Genital Dermatoses

incubated at 33°C in high humidity with 5% carbon dioxide for a minimum of 48-72 hours.

Culture media includes:
- Gonococci (GC) agar supplemented with 1-2% bovine hemoglobin, 5% fetal calf-serum, 1% isovitalex, and 3 mg/L vancomycin
- Mueller-Hinton agar enriched with 5% chocolatized horse blood, isovitalex, and 3 mg/L vancomycin.

- Detection of nucleic acid [deoxyribonucleic acid (DNA)] by amplification techniques, such as polymerase chain reaction (PCR)
- Microscopy of a gram-stained smear (or other stains) of material from the ulcer base or of pus aspirate from the bubo: demonstration of characteristic gram-negative coccobacilli
- Other diagnostic tests have included various antigen-detection techniques involving immunofluorescence or radio-isotopic probes. The detection of antibody to *H. ducreyi* as a marker of chancroid has been useful in a number of epidemiological studies, using enzyme-linked immunoassays (EIAs). In addition, serological screening for syphilis and HIV should be offered. Biopsy of lymph nodes may be required to exclude neoplasia.

Treatment

Successful treatment of chancroid should cure infection, resolve clinical symptoms, and prevent transmission to sexual partners.

Recommended Regimens

- Azithromycin 1 g orally in a single dose or
- Ceftriaxone 250 mg intramuscularly in a single dose or
- Ciprofloxacin 500 mg orally in a single dose or
- Ciprofloxacin 500 mg orally two times a day for 3 days or
- Erythromycin base 500 mg orally four times a day for 7 days.

Azithromycin and ceftriaxone offer the advantage of single-dose therapy. They have excellent in vitro activity against *H. ducreyi*. The safety of azithromycin for pregnant and lactating women has not been established. Ciprofloxacin is contraindicated for pregnant and lactating women, children, and adolescents less than 18 years of age. The erythromycin or ceftriaxone regimens should be used. No adverse effects of chancroid on pregnancy outcome or on the fetus have been reported.

The classic strategy has been to needle-aspirate fluctuant buboes from adjacent healthy skin. The procedure is simpler and safer than incision, which is prone to complications (sinus formations). This procedure should always be performed under effective antibiotic cover.

Patients should be re-examined 3–7 days after initiation of therapy. If treatment is successful, ulcers improve symptomatically within 3 days and substantial re-epithelialization occurs within 7 days after onset of therapy. The time required for complete healing is related to the size of the ulcer (and perhaps HIV-related immunosuppression); large ulcers may require more than 2 weeks.

Persons who have had sexual contact with a patient who has chancroid within the 10 days before onset of the patient's symptoms should be examined, and treated even in the absence of symptoms, as asymptomatic carriage of *H. ducreyi* has been proven to occur.

GRANULOMA INGUINALE (DONOVANOSIS)

Granuloma inguinale, granuloma venereum, ulcerating granuloma of the pudendum, or groin ulceration, as it has been variously designated, is a granulative ulceration of the inguinal region, which may involve the external genitals, perineum, anus, and inner surface of the thighs. The granuloma inguinale lesion is attributed to infection by *Calymmatobacterium granulomatis*, a gram-negative rod.

Calymmatobacterium granulomatis appears as bipolar-staining intracellular inclusions; this organism is a coccobacillus measuring 0.5–1.5 µm wide and 1.0 µm long, with rounded ends. Chromatin condensations at the extremities form safety pins, when stained with Giemsa or Wright stains. These bipolar, safety-pin shaped rods in the cytoplasm of macrophages are the Donovan bodies (DB).

Genital Dermatoses

Sexual contact is believed to be a central part of transmission. Transmission to children is also possible during natural vaginal birth. Although the exact incubation period for granuloma inguinale is unknown, it ranges from a day to a year, with the median time being 50 days.

Clinical Features

The four main types of cutaneous lesions are as follows:
1. *Nodular:* The initial granuloma inguinale lesion is a papule or nodule that arises at the site of inoculation. The nodule is soft, often pruritic and erythematous, and eventually ulcerates. A nodule may be mistaken for a lymph node (i.e., pseudobubo).
2. *Ulcerovegetative (most common):* These granuloma inguinale lesions develop from nodular lesions and consist of large, usually painless, expanding, and suppurative ulcers. The ulcers have clean, friable bases with distinct, raised, rolled margins and have a tendency to bleed easily. The ulcers are "beefy red" and slowly expand centrifugally, eventually becoming more granulomatous with serpiginous borders. They are commonly located in the skin folds, and autoinoculation is a common feature, resulting in lesions on adjacent skin.
3. *Cicatricial:* Dry ulcers evolve into cicatricial plaques and may be associated with lymphedema.
4. *Hypertrophic or verrucous (relatively rare):* This is a proliferative reaction, with the formation of large vegetating masses.

Elephantiasis like swelling of the external genitalia is a frequent complication and is found most often in infected females in the late stage of granuloma inguinale. The most common locations of granuloma inguinale lesions in men are the sulcocoronal and balanopreputial regions, as well as the anus. In women, granuloma inguinale lesions occur on the labia minora, the mons veneris, the fourchette, and/or the cervix. Cervical involvement occurs in 10% of cases. Extragenital involvement occurs in 6% of granuloma inguinale cases. Autoinoculation or direct extension may lead to involvement of the lips, oral or gastrointestinal mucosa, scalp, abdomen, arms, legs, and bones.

Diagnosis

The demonstration of DB in tissue smears is the simple, most reliable, and useful diagnostic measure. A cotton swab is gently rolled over the ulcer so as not to cause bleeding. The swab is then rolled over a glass slide. The slide is allowed to air dry and is then stained with Giemsa stain or to demonstrate DB. Alternatively, a small piece of tissue should be obtained from the ulcer edge or base via punch biopsy, or curettage and the tissue is crushed between two glass slides, separated, and then air dried. A Wright-Giemsa, Warthin-Starry, toluidine blue or Leishman stain may be used to demonstrate the DB.

Tissue smears may be negative for DB in early and late lesions. However, they should be repeated on atleast three consecutive days before being considered negative. Fine needle aspiration cytological smears stained with Giemsa or Leishman stain from pseudobubo lesions are helpful for quick diagnosis.

In suspected cases, where DB cannot be demonstrated in tissue smears, a biopsy can be obtained from the active edge of the ulcer to confirm diagnosis. Special stains such as Giemsa and hematoxylin and eosin are helpful to demonstrate DB in histological sections.

It is essential to perform body imaging and radiographic studies, if metastatic or systemic dissemination with bone involvement is suspected as an extragenital manifestation. Culture of *Klebsiella granulomatis* from feces has been reported using a monocyte co-culture system.

Polymerase chain reaction techniques may be more sensitive; however, they are currently only used for scientific research.

Treatment

All patients with active lesions shown to contain DB should receive antimicrobial treatment. Patients from areas endemic for donovanosis with a clinical diagnosis of the disease should be given presumptive treatment. Various drugs found to be effective in the treatment of donovanosis in prospective studies are are given in Table 1.

TABLE 1: Various drugs found to be effective in the treatment of donovanosis

Drugs	Route	Dosage
Streptomycin	Intramuscularly	2 g twice daily for 5 days
Chloramphenicol	Oral	500 mg four times daily for 14 days
Cotrimoxazole DS	Oral	1 tab twice daily for 14 days
Tetracycline	Oral	500 mg four times daily for 14 days
Doxycycline	Oral	100 mg twice daily for 14 days
Erythromycin	Oral	500 mg four times daily for 14 days
Norfloxacin	Oral	400 mg twice daily for 14 days
Ciprofloxacin	Oral	500 mg twice daily for 14 days
Azithromycin	Oral	500 mg daily for 7 days
Ceftriaxone	Intramuscularly	1 g for 7 days

Any person with a history of unprotected sexual contact with a patient with active donovanosis or within 40 days before the onset of lesions should be assessed clinically for evidence of infection and offered treatment. Patients should be followed until symptoms have resolved. The lesion should be monitored clinically or via serial biopsies to look for DB. In advanced disease, with vast tissue obliteration and scarring, surgery may be required.

LYMPHOGRANULOMA VENEREUM

Lymphogranuloma venereum (LGV) is caused by serovars L1, L2, and L3 of the obligate intracellular bacterium *Chlamydia trachomatis (C. trachomatis)*. These LGV strains are more virulent in animal models than the more prevalent serovars A–K of *C. trachomatis*, and more invasive in humans. Whereas serovars A–K are largely confined to mucosal columnar epithelial surfaces of the genital tract and eye, the LGV serovars infect predominantly monocytes and macrophages, pass through the epithelial surface to regional lymph nodes, and may cause disseminated infection.

Clinical Features

The clinical course of LGV can be divided into three stages. The primary stage involves the site of inoculation; the secondary stage the regional lymph nodes and sometimes the anorectum; and late sequelae, affecting the genitals and/or rectum, comprise the tertiary stage.

1. *Primary Stage:* After an incubation period of 3–30 days, a small, painless papule, which may ulcerate, appears at the site of inoculation (usually the prepuce or glans in men, and the vulva, vaginal wall or occasionally, cervix in women). The primary lesion is self-limiting. It may not always occur, and may pass unnoticed by the patient.
2. *Secondary Stage:* The secondary stage occurs some weeks after the primary lesion. It may chiefly involve the inguinal lymph nodes or the anus and rectum. The inguinal form is more common in men, since the lymphatic drainage of the vagina and cervix is to the retroperitoneal rather than the inguinal lymph nodes. Proctitis due to LGV is more common in women and in men who practice receptive anal intercourse, and is thought to be due to direct inoculation.

    The cardinal feature of the inguinal form of LGV is the presence of painful inguinal and/or femoral lymphadenopathy, which is usually unilateral. The presence of adenopathy above and below the inguinal ligament gives rise to the "groove sign" once believed to be pathognomonic for LGV, in 10–20% of cases. Enlarged lymph nodes are usually firm, and biopsy reveals small discrete areas of necrosis surrounded by proliferating epithelioid and endothelial cells. These areas of necrosis may enlarge to form stellate abscesses, which may coalesce and break down to form discharging sinuses, though this phenomenon occurs in less than one-third of patients, and is more common in chancroid.

    Extragenital inoculation can give rise to lymphadenopathy outside the inguinal region.

    Anorectal involvement in early LGV was described many years ago, predominantly in women and homosexual men, presenting with an acute hemorrhagic proctitis. Patients present

with rectal pain and bleeding, often with pronounced systemic features (fever, chills, and weight loss). Proctoscopy reveals a granular or ulcerative proctitis, resembling ulcerative colitis, confined to the distal 10 cm of the anorectal canal.
3. *Tertiary Stage:* Chronic inflammatory lesions caused by *C. trachomatis* often lead to scarring in both the eye and genital tract. In chronic untreated LGV, fibrosis can lead to lymphatic obstruction, causing elephantiasis of the genitalia in either sex, and rectal involvement can lead to the formation of strictures and fistulae. These conditions are more common in women, and can give rise to the syndrome of esthiomene (Greek: "Eating away"), with widespread destruction of the external genitalia.

Differential Diagnosis

Lymphogranuloma venereum may present as a genital ulcer or as inguinal lymphadenopathy (usually painful) without evidence of genital ulceration. The differential diagnosis of sexually acquired genital ulceration includes chancroid, herpes, syphilis, and donovanosis (granuloma inguinale). The differential diagnosis of inguinal adenopathy includes chancroid, herpes, and syphilis, although there is usually a genital ulcer or at least a history of an ulcer in these conditions. Unilateral inguinal or femoral lymphadenopathy should prompt a careful search for septic lesions of the leg or the foot. Chronic sinus formation in the inguinal region may be due to tuberculosis of the lumbar spine, and bubonic plague should be considered in the acutely ill patient with inguinal lymphadenopathy in endemic areas.

Diagnosis

In the past, LGV was diagnosed by the Frei skin test, a test of delayed type hypersensitivity to chlamydial antigens, similar to the tuberculin test. This test was not as sensitive as serology, and probably resulted in many false positives. The diagnosis of LGV now depends on serology or on the identification of *C trachomatis* in appropriate clinical samples. When available, histopathological examination of biopsy specimens can also support the diagnosis. The complement fixation test has been used for many years to diagnose chlamydial infections. The microimmunofluorescence (MIF) test can distinguish between infections with different chlamydial species, but has not been much used in routine clinical practice, since it requires a fluorescent microscope and a skilled technologist trained in the technique. *C. trachomatis* can be identified in bubo fluid following aspiration, or in ulcer material. In contrast with chancroid, buboes of which contain large amounts of pus, the buboes of LGV may contain only small amounts of thin milky fluid, and it may be necessary to inject 2-5 mL of sterile saline to obtain any fluid by aspiration. *C. trachomatis* can be isolated in tissue culture, using HeLa 229 or McCoy cell lines, but this technique is not widely available.

Commercially available EIAs, which detect chlamydial antigens [usually lipopolysaccharide (LPS)] are widely used to diagnose urethral and cervical infection with *C. trachomatis* serovars D-K, but have not been evaluated for the diagnosis of LGV. DNA amplification assays—for example, PCR or ligase chain reaction (LCR), which detects *Chlamydia* specific genomic or plasmid DNA, are the most sensitive tests available for the diagnosis of genital *C. trachomatis* infection.

Treatment

Recommended treatment for both bubonic and anogenital LGV is tetracycline 500 mg four times daily for 14 days or doxycycline 100 mg twice daily for 14 days, or erythromycin 500 mg four times daily for 14 days. Erythromycin should be given to pregnant women, in whom tetracyclines are contraindicated. Patients with advanced disease may require treatment for more than 14 days. Large collections of pus should be aspirated, using a lateral approach through normal skin. Late complications such as rectal stricture may be improved by antibiotic treatment, which reduces the inflammatory component, but does not correct damage due to fibrosis. Rectovaginal fistula, bowel obstruction, and esthiomene require surgical correction under antibiotic cover.

BACTERIAL VAGINOSIS

Bacterial vaginosis (BV), a polymicrobial syndrome characterized by an imbalance of the ordinary vaginal microbiota, results from the substitution of high concentration, the hydrogen peroxide (H_2O_2) producing *Lactobacillus* spp. for nondominant or exogenous bacteria. The condition is present in approximately 30% of the women of child-bearing age. *Gardnerella vaginalis* is a facultative anaerobic, fastidious β-hemolytic, immobile, encapsulated, pleomorphic, and Gram-variable.

The physiologic pH of the vagina ranges from 3.8 to 4.5. By using glycogen from the vaginal epithelium as substrate, lactobacilli produce organic acids, thus keeping the vaginal pH below 4.5. This acid environment partially or fully inhibits the development of most bacteria from both, the digestive tract and the environment. This is, therefore, a very efficient mechanism of mucosal protection. Changes in some metabolic factors may affect the microbiological balance in this syndrome. Glucose from vaginal glycogen is no longer degraded into lactic acid by H_2O_2-producing lactobacilli, being transformed instead into fatty acids by anaerobic bacteria. These fatty acids increase vaginal pH over 4.5, thus creating an unfavorable milieu for lactobacilli growth, while favorable to the growth of potentially pathogenic bacteria, closing a cycle that allows for the development of BV. Amino acid degradation, through anaerobic bacteria-related enzymatic mechanisms, leads to the production of different compounds, biogenic amines or polyamines among them. Lysine and ornithine decarboxylation produces cadaverine and putrescine, respectively, while histidine degradation produces histamine. High levels of biogenic amines, such as putrescine, cadaverine, and trimethylamine have been found in vaginal secretions of women with BV.

Some risk factors seem to be related to BV, such as age, ethnicity, smoking, vaginal douches, intrauterine devices (IUD), and sexual behavior.

Clinical manifestations and diagnosis of BV may be symptomatic or asymptomatic. Symptomatic BV is characterized by a copious,

Sexually Transmitted Infection Affecting the Genitalia

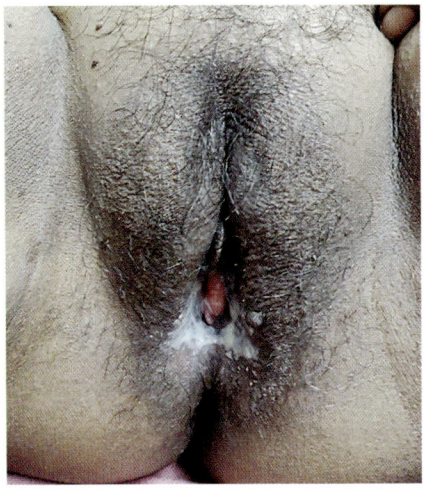

Figure 7: Bacterial vaginosis showing greyish discharge and erythema of the vulva

thin, homogeneous, milky, foul-smelling vaginal flow, which is exacerbated after intercourse without condom use and menstruation (Fig. 7). When some drops of 10% potassium hydroxide (KOH) are added to a vaginal secretion preparation (KOH wet mount-Whiff test), a rotten-fish odor, caused by the presence of volatile biogenic amines, such as putrescine, cadaverine, and trimethylamine can be perceived. Vaginal pH is over 4.5, and microscopic examination of vaginal flow shows clue-cells, exfoliated vaginal or ectocervical cells superficially covered with *G. vaginalis*, *Bacteroides* spp., and *Mobiluncus* spp.

Amsel criteria are generally used in clinical practice for diagnosing both symptomatic and asymptomatic BV. At least three of the four criteria should be met:
1. Copious, thin, homogeneous, milky vaginal discharge
2. Rotten-fish odor due to the release of volatile amines on Whiff test
3. Vaginal pH more than 4.5, and
4. Identification of bacteria-covered epithelial cells (clue-cells) under light microscopy.

Even without vaginal discharge, asymptomatic BV can be easily diagnosed when criteria 2, 3, and 4 are met.

Nugent score is now the accepted gold standard for BV diagnosis. According to the Nugent method, Gram-stained smears are used for identification, classification, and quantification of the following bacterial morphotypes: *Lactobacillus* spp. (Gram-positive bacilli), *G. vaginalis* and *Bacteroides* spp. (Gram-negative or Gram-variable cocobacilli), and *Mobiluncus* spp. (curved Gram-negative bacilli). Each morphotype is quantified and scored according to a 0–10 scale, and any value equal to or greater than 7 being considered positive for BV.

Another widely used method for diagnosing BV in clinical practice is the Papanicolaou-stained smear technique in suggestive cases; pathologists also report the presence of clue cells in these smears.

Specific recommendations for treatment of BV:
- For nonpregnant women, the first option includes oral metronidazole 400–600 mg, twice a day for 7 days and the second option includes oral metronidazole (2 g) in a single dose, or intravaginal metronidazole 7.5% twice a day for 5 days, or oral clindamycin 300 mg, twice a day for 7 days or intravaginal clindamycin 2% once a day for 7 days
- For pregnant women after the first trimester and during breastfeeding, oral metronidazole 250–400 mg, three times a day for 7 days or clindamycin 300 mg, twice a day for 7 days.

Tinidazole was the first new antibiotic approved for BV treatment in the last 20 years. This second generation of nitroimidazoles has also been approved for treatment of trichomoniasis, being the only oral agent approved for both conditions. It's half-life is twice as long as that of metronidazole and side effects is observed in half as many patients in comparison with the latter.

TRICHOMONIASIS

Trichomonas vaginalis (TV), a parasitic protozoan, is the etiologic agent of trichomoniasis, a STD of worldwide importance.

Trichomoniasis is the most common nonviral STD, and it is associated with many perinatal complications, male and female genitourinary tract infections, and an increased incidence of HIV transmission.

Trichomonas vaginalis is a parasitic protozoan flagellate, and organisms vary in size but are usually around 10 μm in length and 7 μm in width. It usually has an oval or pear-like shape, but can assume an amoeboid form when attached to vaginal epithelial cells. TV has a total of five flagella, four of which are located at its anterior portion. The fifth flagellum is incorporated within the undulating membrane. The anaerobic parasite can only exist as a trophozoite and lacks a cystic stage, reproducing by longitudinal binary fission. Growth is optimized at 37°C at pH 6.0–6.3, but can survive at up to pH 7. Structure of *T. vaginalis* is given in Fig. 8.

It commonly spreads through sexual contact with vaginal or urethral discharges of infected persons. Nonsexual transmission is rare but has been observed in cases involving contaminated douche nozzles, moist wash-clothes, specula, or toilet seats.

In women, symptoms of infection include vaginal secretion that is scanty and mixed with mucous, malodorous discharge that is

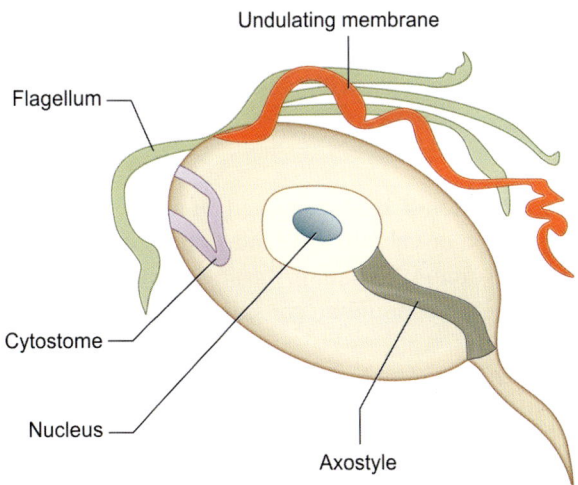

Figure 8: Structure of *Trichomonas vaginalis*

Genital Dermatoses

frothy, yellow or green, mucopurulent, and copious. The protozoan can be found in the vagina, cervix, bladder, Bartholin's, Skene's, and periurethral glands. Complications may result in cervical erosion, cervical cancer, infertility, adnexitis, pyosalpinx, and endometritis. Premature rupture of the placental membranes can occur in pregnant women, resulting in premature birth and low-birth weight. Acute infections are characterized by severe pruritus, vaginitis, vulvitis with dysuria and dyspareunia, and hemorrhagic spots on the mucosa (in 2% of patients) which results in colpitis macularis or petechiae (strawberry cervix). In females, 50% of cases are asymptomatic. Infection can persist for long periods of time in the urogenital tract of women. 25-50% are asymptomatic for the first 6 months of infection, and organisms can survive indefinitely in the lower urogenital tract, if left untreated.

Prevalence is lower in men, and infection is often asymptomatic. Infection in men can be present in the prostate, seminal vesicles, and epididymis. Complications are rare, but can potentially lead to genitourinary inflammation disease, sterility, scanty, clear to mucopurulent discharge, dysuria, nongonococcal urethritis, prostatitis, balanoposthitis, epididymitis, and urethral disease. Infection is usually mild with no symptoms, thus making men potential carriers. Spontaneous resolution of infection is common as the oxidative nature of the male genital tract is speculated to be inhibitory to pathogenic factors of infection, which usually remains for 10 days or less.

Diagnosis

Testing for TV should be undertaken in women complaining of vaginal discharge or vulvitis, or found to have evidence of vulvitis, and/or vaginitis on examination. Testing in men is recommended for TV contacts, and should be considered in those with persistent urethritis.

Sites Sampled

Females
- Swab taken from the posterior fornix at the time of speculum examination

- Urine has been used for evaluation with some nucleic acid amplification tests (NAATs).

Males
- Urethral culture or culture of first-void urine will diagnose 60–80% cases, sampling both sites simultaneously will significantly increase the diagnostic rate using microscopy or culture.

Laboratory Investigations

Microscopy: Detection of motile trichomonads by light-field microscopy can be achieved by collection of vaginal discharge using a swab or loop, which is then mixed with a small drop of saline on a glass slide and a coverslip placed on top. The wet preparation should be read within 10 minutes of collection, as the trichomonads will quickly loose motility and be more difficult to identify. The slide should be scanned, firstly at low magnification (x100), and then at a higher magnification (x400) to confirm the morphology of any trichomonads and to visualize the flagella. Microscopy as a diagnostic aid for TV has the advantage that it can be performed near to the patient and in a clinic setting. The sensitivity is highest in women presenting with vaginal discharge and a visualization of motile trichomonads in these women indicates the presence of infection. However, the sensitivity is reported to be as low as 45–60% in women in some studies and lower in men, and so a negative result should be interpreted with caution. The specificity with trained personnel is high.

Culture: Culture of TV has a higher sensitivity compared to microscopy and can detect TV in men. A commercially available culture system (InPouch TV) offers many advantages over previous culture media, such as Diamond's medium. Once inoculated the pouches can be transferred to the laboratory for incubation and the entire pouch read microscopically each day for 5 days, negating the need to prepare wet preparations every day that only sample portion of the culture medium. Culture was considered "the gold standard" but the molecular testing has proven to have a higher sensitivity.

Molecular detection: Nucleic acid amplification tests offer the highest sensitivity for the detection of TV. They should be the test of choice where resources allow and are becoming the current "gold standard".

In-house PCRs have shown increased sensitivity in comparison to both microscopy and culture, which has been found to be even greater using the commercial Food and Drug Administration (FDA) approved platform which can detect TV DNA in vaginal or endocervical swabs and in urine samples from women and men with sensitivities of 88–97% and specificities of 98–99%.

Management

General advice: Sexual partners should be treated simultaneously. Patients should be advised to avoid sexual intercourse for at least 1 week until they and their partners have completed treatment.

Treatment

Systemic antibiotic therapy is required to affect a permanent cure due to the high frequency of infection of the urethra and paraurethral glands in females. A cochrane review has found that almost any nitroimidazole drug given as a single dose or over a longer period results in parasitological cure in more than 90% of cases. Oral single dose treatment with any nitroimidazole seems to be effective in achieving short-term parasitological cure, but is associated with more frequent side effects than either longer oral or intravaginal treatment. Intravaginal treatment showed parasitological cure rates around 50%, which is unacceptably low. There is a spontaneous cure rate in the order of 20–25%.

Recommended Regimes
- Metronidazole 2 g orally in a single dose or
- Metronidazole 400–500 mg twice daily for 5–7 days.

Alternative Regimen
- Tinidazole 2 g orally in a single dose. Tinidazole has similar activity to metronidazole but is more expensive.

Pregnancy and Breast Feeding

Metronidazole is likely to cure trichomoniasis, but it is not known whether this treatment will have any effect on pregnancy outcomes.

Meta-analyses have concluded that there is no evidence of teratogenicity from the use of metronidazole in women during the first trimester of pregnancy. Metronidazole can be used in all stages of pregnancy and during breastfeeding. Symptomatic women should be treated at diagnosis, although some clinicians have preferred to defer treatment until the second trimester. Metronidazole enters breast milk and may affect its taste. The manufacturers recommend avoiding high doses, if breastfeeding or if using a single dose of metronidazole, breastfeeding should be discontinued for 12–24 hours to reduce infant exposure.

Tinidazole is pregnancy category C (animal studies have demonstrated an adverse event, and no adequate, well-controlled studies in pregnant women have been conducted), and it's safety in pregnant women has not been well-evaluated. The manufacturer states that the use of tinidazole in the first trimester is contraindicated.

Treatment protocol for nonresponse to standard TV therapy (having excluded reinfection and nonadherence):
- Repeat course of 7-days standard therapy

Metronidazole 400–500 mg twice daily for 7 days; in those who failed to respond to a first course of treatment, 40% responded to a repeat course of standard treatment.

For patients failing, this second regimen:
- Higher dose course of nitroimidazole
- Metronidazole or tinidazole 2 g daily for 5–7 days or
- Metronidazole 800 mg three times daily for 7 days, in those who failed to respond to a second course of treatment, 70% responded to a higher dose course of metronidazole.

For those failing this third regimen, resistance testing should be performed, if available as improved outcomes were reported with a treatment protocol guided by the results of a resistance test. If resistance testing is not available, high-dose tinidazole regimens are recommended.
- Very high-dose course of tinidazole
- Tinidazole 1 g twice or three times daily, or 2 g twice daily for 14 days + or − intravaginal tinidazole 500 mg twice daily for 14 days.

If very high-dose tinidazole has been unsuccessful, it is difficult to recommend one specific further treatment. Treatment of such cases can be a therapeutic challenge as treatment options are limited with little evidence to support them. The largest published case series have been with intravaginal paromomycin and intravaginal furazolidone. There are anecdotal reports of treatment success with a number of other treatments. The reports are based on success in one or two women who had usually received a wide variety of prior treatments. Consequently for each successful anecdote, there are a number of reports of treatment failure.

Other treatments with some reported success are:
- Paromomycin intravaginally 250 mg once or twice daily for 14 days: 56–58% cure rate reported
- Furazolidone intravaginally 100 mg twice daily for 12–14 days: 33% cure rate reported
- Acetarsol pessaries 500 mg nocte for 2 weeks
- 6% nonoxynol-9 pessaries nightly for 2 weeks.

SYPHILIS

Syphilis is primarily a sexually transmitted infection (STI). Syphilis can also be acquired through congenital transmission to the newborn and blood transfusion, but these are much less common. It is a systemic disease caused by the spirochete *Treponema pallidum (T. pallidum)* subspecies *pallidum*. This is one of the clinically important spirochetes and is related to such agents as *Borrelia burgdorferi* (the cause of Lyme disease) and *Leptospira* (the cause of leptospirosis). Syphilis occurs exclusively in humans; there is no animal reservoir. The infection can be classified as congenital (transmitted from mother to child in utero) or acquired (through sex or blood transfusion).

Acquired syphilis is divided into early and late syphilis. Early syphilis comprises the primary, secondary, and early latent stages. Late syphilis refers to late latent syphilis, gummatous, neurological, and cardiovascular syphilis.

Sexually Transmitted Infection Affecting the Genitalia

Case Definitions

- *Incubating Syphilis:* An asymptomatic person with a history of sexual exposure within the past 10–90 days to a partner with a confirmed diagnosis of infectious syphilis; either a reactive serology (nontreponemal and treponemal); at least a fourfold (e.g., 1:8 to 1:32) increase in titre over the last known nontreponemal test. Incubating syphilis is a subset of early latent syphilis
- *Primary Syphilis:* Identification of *T. pallidum* by dark-field microscopy, fluorescent antibody, or equivalent examination of material from a chancre or regional lymph node or presence of one or more typical lesions (chancres), and reactive treponemal serology, regardless of nontreponemal test reactivity in individuals with no previous history of syphilis; or presence of one or more typical lesions (chancres), and at least a fourfold (e.g., 1:8 to 1:32) increase in titre over the last known nontreponemal test in individuals with a past history of syphilis treatment
- *Secondary Syphilis:* Identification of *T. pallidum* by dark-field microscopy, fluorescent antibody, or equivalent examination of mucocutaneous lesions and condyloma lata; or presence of one or more typical mucocutaneous lesions, alopecia, loss of eyelashes and lateral third of eyebrows, iritis, generalized lymphadenopathy, fever, malaise, or splenomegaly; plus either a reactive serology (nontreponemal and treponemal); or at least a fourfold (e.g., 1:8 to 1:32) increase in titre over the last known nontreponemal test
- *Early Latent Syphilis:* An asymptomatic person with reactive serology (nontreponemal and treponemal) who within the past one year had one of the following:
  - Nonreactive serology
  - Symptoms suggestive of primary or secondary syphilis or
  - Exposure to a sexual partner with primary, secondary or early latent syphilis.
- *Late Latent Syphilis:* An asymptomatic person with persistently reactive treponemal serology (regardless of nontreponemal

serology reactivity) who does not meet the criteria for early latent disease and who has not been previously treated for syphilis
- *Neurosyphilis:* Reactive treponemal serology (regardless of nontreponemal serology reactivity) and one of the following:
  - Reactive cerebrospinal fluid (CSF)-venereal disease research laboratory (VDRL) in nonbloody CSF
  - Clinical evidence of neurosyphilis and CSF pleocytosis (particularly lymphocytes) in the absence of other known causes or
  - Clinical evidence of neurosyphilis and elevated CSF protein in the absence of other known causes.

  Neurosyphilis may be seen during primary or secondary syphilis stages and can occur at any time after initial infection.
- *Congenital Syphilis:* Identification of *T. pallidum* by dark-field microscopy, fluorescent antibody, or equivalent examination of material from nasal discharges, skin lesions, placenta or umbilical cord, or autopsy material of a neonate (up to 4 weeks of age); or reactive serology (treponemal and nontreponemal) from venous blood (not cord blood) in an infant or child with clinical, laboratory, or radiographic evidence of congenital syphilis, whose mother is seropositive for syphilis without documented evidence of adequate treatment.

  For a primary chancre, the incubation period is 3 days to 3 months, usually about 3 weeks. Primary syphilis most often presents as a single painless lesion (chancre) that develops at the site of inoculation. The chancre is most commonly found on the external genitalia. These lesions frequently go unnoticed. The ulcer is clean-based with a raised and indurated border. In men, the most common site affected is the penis, more specifically the coronal sulcus and glans (Fig. 9). In women, the most common locations for lesions are the labia majora, labia minora, fourchette, and perineum. Ulcers may also be found on the lip, in the mouth, and on fingers. The chancre usually resolves spontaneously in 1–4 months. Painless, firm regional lymphadenopathy, often associated with genital lesions, is common and occurs in up to

Sexually Transmitted Infection Affecting the Genitalia

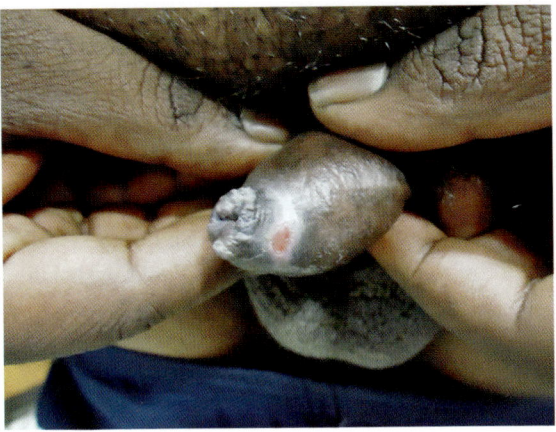

Figure 9: Primary chancre in healing phase after receiving benzathine penicillin.

80% of patients. These clinical findings usually occur about 3 weeks after infection with *T. pallidum*.

Secondary syphilis is most often heralding by a maculopapular rash involving palms and soles, but this stage can include laryngitis, condylomata lata, hepatitis, and meningitis among other manifestations. Condylomata lata are characteristic of secondary syphilis. They are large, fleshy lesions that may form in warm, moist areas, such as the perineum and perianal skin, axillae, and beneath the breasts. These lesions are painless but highly infectious. The original genital chancre is still present in up to 30% of patients with secondary syphilis. Constitutional symptoms such as fevers, muscle aches, and weight loss are also common.

- *Latent Syphilis:* Left untreated, secondary syphilis may progress to a period of subclinical infection. During the latent stage of syphilis, skin lesions resolve and patients are asymptomatic. The only clue for the diagnosis of latent infection is a positive serologic test for syphilis.

Latent syphilis is divided into early latent and late latent syphilis. Patients are classified as having early latent disease, if they are asymptomatic and have acquired the infection within the past year. This stage can be established only in patients who have seroconverted within the past year, who have had symptoms of primary or secondary syphilis within the past year or who have had a sexual partner with primary, secondary, or early latent syphilis within the past year. Patients who do not meet these criteria should be presumed to have late latent syphilis or latent syphilis of unknown duration. A patient with early latent syphilis is considered to be infectious due to the 25% risk of relapse to secondary syphilis. Early latent syphilis is infectious by sexual contact whereas late latent syphilis is not. However, a pregnant woman with late latent syphilis can infect her fetus in utero, and an infection can be transmitted via transfusion of contaminated blood.

- *Tertiary Syphilis:* Tertiary syphilis is a slowly progressive, inflammatory disease that can affect any organ in the body to produce clinical illness 10–30 years after the initial infection. Tertiary syphilis refers to gummatous and cardiovascular syphilis, but not to all neurosyphilis.

  These forms of syphilis are now uncommon:
  - *Gummatous syphilis (late benign syphilis):* Gumma or granulomatous-like lesions are indolent and most commonly found in the skeletal system, skin and mucous membranes, but can develop in any organ. Lesions rarely cause incapacity or death, but when lesions occur in organs like the brain or heart, serious complications occur.
  - *Cardiovascular syphilis:* Cardiovascular syphilis results from destruction of the elastic tissue of the aorta which leads to ascending aortitis and the formation of aneurysms that rarely rupture. The ascending aorta is most often affected, with the potential complications of valve insufficiency and coronary artery stenosis. Approximately, 11% of untreated patients progress to cardiovascular syphilis.
  - *Neurosyphilis:* Central nervous system (CNS) disease can occur during any stage of syphilis. A patient who has clinical

evidence of neurologic involvement with syphilis (e.g., cognitive dysfunction, motor or sensory deficits, ophthalmic or auditory symptoms, cranial nerve palsies, and symptoms or signs of meningitis) should have a CSF examination. Neurosyphilis is divided into early (acute) neurosyphilis and late (chronic) neurosyphilis. Both early and late neurosyphilis can be divided into asymptomatic and symptomatic phases. The symptomatic phase of late neurosyphilis is further distinguished as meningovascular or parenchymatous neurosyphilis. Clinical overlap with combinations of meningovascular and parenchymatous features are common as this form of chronic meningitis involves every portion of the CNS.

Asymptomatic neurosyphilis occurs in up to 40% of patients. It is defined as patients who have no clinical manifestations of neurologic involvement but who have one or more of the following CSF abnormalities: elevated white blood cells (WBC) count, elevated protein concentration, a decreased glucose concentration, or a positive nontreponemal test (e.g., VDRL). Rapid plasma reagin (RPR) is not recommended for CSF testing.

Syphilis and Pregnancy

Syphilis can be transmitted transplacentally to the fetus at all stages during the course of untreated maternal disease from incubating syphilis to primary, secondary, tertiary, and latent disease. Syphilis can also be transmitted during passage through the birth canal when the newborn infant contacts a genital lesion. Breastfeeding does not result in transmission of syphilis unless an infectious lesion is present on the breast. Pregnancy has no known effect on the clinical course of syphilis. The rate of vertical transmission in untreated women is 70-100% in primary syphilis, 40% for early latent syphilis, and 10% for latent disease. The longer the interval between infection and pregnancy, the more benign is the outcome in the infant.

All pregnant women should be screened for syphilis (with a nontreponemal test) and other STIs (including HIV) on their first prenatal visit. High seroconversion rates for both syphilis and HIV in high-risk populations during pregnancy has led some experts to suggest repeat screening of women during late pregnancy and delivery.

Syphilis in pregnancy can cause widespread complications for both the infected mother and fetus. At least two-thirds of all babies born to untreated women with syphilis are infected. If evidence of syphilis is present, treatment should be initiated immediately according to the stage of the disease. Efficacy of syphilis treatment in pregnancy considers resolution of maternal infection and prevention of congenital syphilis.

Clinical manifestations of congenital syphilis are divided into early (appear within the first 2 years of life) and late (after first 2 years of life) stages. Late congenital syphilis usually manifests near puberty. Most clinical signs of early congenital syphilis develop within the first 3 months of life. Snuffles or persistent rhinitis is one of the earliest clinical manifestations occurring in 4–22% of infants. The nasal discharge may be profuse, purulent, or blood tinged and is highly infectious. Hepatomegaly with or without splenomegaly occurs in 33–100% of patients. Asymptomatic CNS involvement manifesting in CSF abnormalities of lymphocytosis, elevated protein levels, and positive serologic tests occur in up to 80% of infected infants. Symptomatic neurosyphilis develops rarely. Bone lesions develop within 8 months of birth in early congenital syphilis. Late manifestations of congenital syphilis include Hutchinson's triad of interstitial keratitis; peg-shaped upper incisors, and 8th cranial nerve deafness. The hearing loss can be sudden and usually occurs at 8–10 years of age.

Human Immunodeficiency Virus and Syphilis

Many regions in the tropics have high prevalence of both HIV infection and syphilis. Syphilis can mimic HIV infection and vice versa: Chancre versus chronic mucocutaneous anogenital herpes in acquired immune deficiency syndrome (AIDS), secondary syphilis versus primary HIV infection and neurosyphilis versus neurological complications of HIV infection. HIV infection can lead to larger or more numerous chancres, accelerated ulcerating secondary syphilis, frequent ocular syphilis, faster progression to late syphilis, such as neurosyphilis and gummatous syphilis; the former have been reported mainly in those treated for early syphilis with single dose benzathine penicillin. Although serological tests in HIV-positive patients is generally performed in the same way as in immunocompetent patients, it can occasionally behave unpredictably—for example, delayed positive serological tests in secondary syphilis. Biological false positives for cardiolipin tests (VDRL, RPR) and prozone phenomenon can also occur in HIV infection.

Diagnosis

Although *T. pallidum* cannot be grown in culture, there are many tests for the direct and indirect diagnosis of syphilis. Still, there is no single optimal test. Direct diagnostic methods include the detection of *T. pallidum* by microscopic examination of fluid or smears from lesions and histological examination of tissues or nucleic acid amplification methods such as PCR. Indirect diagnosis is based on serological tests for the detection of antibodies. Serological tests fall into two categories: nontreponemal tests for screening, and treponemal tests for confirmation. All nontreponemal tests measure both immunoglobulin IgG and IgM antiphospholipid antibodies formed by the host in response to lipoidal material, released by damaged host cells early in infection and lipid from the cell surfaces of the treponeme itself. All treponemal tests use *T. pallidum* or its components as the antigen. If lesion exudate or tissue is available, direct examination is performed, followed by a nontreponemal serology test. A reactive nontreponemal test is then confirmed by a treponemal test. A confirmed serological test result is indicative of the presence of treponemal antibodies but does not indicate the stage of disease, and depending on the test, may not differentiate between past and current infection. Despite their shortcomings and the complexity of interpretation, serological tests are the mainstay in the diagnosis and follow-up of syphilis. Latent syphilis can only be diagnosed by serological tests.

Specimen of Choice

For direct examination, exudates from lesions of primary, secondary, and early congenital syphilis are the most useful. It is important to collect clear, serous fluid free of erythrocytes, tissue debris, and other organisms. Gentle abrasion of lesions may be necessary to express clear, serous fluid. Lesions should be cleansed with saline or water before collecting the specimen. This is especially important when collecting specimens from areas such as under the prepuce, where nonpathogenic treponemes may be present. For dark-field microscopy, the fluid should be collected on a slide, covered with a coverslip, and examined within 20 minutes. For direct fluorescent antibody testing, a smear should be made on a slide and then air dried.

While plasma can be used in some nontreponemal serological tests, serum is the specimen of choice for both nontreponemal and treponemal serological tests. CSF testing is indicated in congenital and tertiary syphilis and when neurological symptoms are present. Blood contamination of CSF must be avoided because it may lead to false-positive CSF results. In congenital syphilis, venous samples from the mother and the child should be tested.

Tests for Direct Detection of Treponema pallidum

Dark-field microscopy: This method still remains one of the simplest and most reliable for the direct detection of *T. pallidum*. Exudates and fluids from lesions are examined as a wet mount using dark-field microscopy. The identification of *T. pallidum* is based on the characteristic morphology and motility of the spirochete. This method is suitable when the lesions are moist, and the examination can be done immediately after specimen collection. During the primary stage, serous fluid from the lesion contains numerous treponemes and therefore, this approach is particularly useful in patients with immunodeficiency or in early syphilis when antibodies are not yet detectable. However, this technique requires a trained, experienced person.

Direct fluorescent antibody test for Treponema pallidum: The direct fluorescent antibody test for *T. pallidum* is easier to perform than dark-field microscopy. It detects antigen and, thus, does not require the presence of motile treponemes. It is the most specific test for the diagnosis of syphilis, when lesions are present. This test uses fluorescein isothiocyanate-labeled antibody specific to pathogenic treponemes, and therefore is suitable for the examination of specimens from oral and rectal lesions. However, this test does not differentiate between *T. pallidum* and other pathogenic treponemes causing yaws, endemic syphilis, and pinta.

Nucleic acid amplification methods: A number of PCR-based methods have been developed for the detection of *T. pallidum* in clinical specimens. Although, these methods are not standardized, they have been found to be highly sensitive, able to detect as low as one to ten organisms per specimen with high specificity. These methods are also the most practical in certain settings. PCR, undoubtedly, holds promise as a test of choice for congenital syphilis, neurosyphilis, and early primary syphilis when traditional tests have limited sensitivity. This method could be used to monitor treatment, and there is also potential to use it to differentiate new infections from old infections.

Nontreponemal Serological Tests

Centers for Disease Control and Prevention approved standard tests, including the VDRL slide test, the rapid plasma reagin (RPR) card test, the unheated serum reagin (USR) test, and the toluidine red unheated serum test (TRUST). Nontreponemal tests are rapid, simple, and inexpensive. They are the only tests recommended to monitor the course of disease during and after treatment. Nontreponemal tests can also serve to detect reinfection. The main limitations of nontreponemal tests are their reduced sensitivity in primary syphilis and late latent syphilis, false-positive results due to cross-reactivity, and the potential for false-negative results due to prozone reactions. Prozone reactions are false-negative reactions that occur due to interference by high concentrations of target antibodies in a specimen. The disproportionate antibody-to-antigen ratio results in a "rough" nonreactive or a very weakly reactive reaction. Such specimens will give a clearly positive reaction when diluted and retested, a process that brings the antibody-to-antigen ratio within the optimal range.

Venereal Disease Research Laboratory, Rapid Plasma Reagin, Unheated Serum Reagin, and Toluidine Red Unheated Serum Tests

The VDRL and USR tests are microflocculation tests and are read under a microscope. A disadvantage of the VDRL test is that the antigen suspension must be prepared fresh daily, whereas the USR test uses a stabilized antigen. However, the VDRL test is the only nontreponemal test that can be used to test CSF due to the limited sensitivity and specificity of the other nontreponemal tests. The RPR and TRUST tests are macroscopic flocculation tests and require no microscope. The RPR test uses a stabilized suspension of VDRL antigen to which charcoal particles are added to aid in the visualization of the test reaction. The RPR test is one of the most commonly used nontreponemal tests, and is a simplified version of the VDRL test. In the TRUST test, particles of toluidine red are used in place of the charcoal particles of the RPR test. Each of the above tests can be used as a quantitative test. Quantitative tests allow for the establishment of a baseline titre, which allows evaluation of recent infection and response to treatment. This also allows for the detection of reinfection or relapse in persons with a persistently reactive titre.

Treponemal Serological Tests

Treponemal tests may remain reactive for years with or without treatment, and treponemal test antibody titres correlate poorly with disease activity. Therefore, treponemal tests should not be used to evaluate response to therapy, relapse, or reinfection in previously treated patients. Also, treponemal tests do not differentiate venereal syphilis from endemic syphilis (yaws and pinta). Treponemal tests are used mainly as confirmatory tests to verify reactivity in nontreponemal tests. However, in populations of low disease prevalence, treponemal tests can be used for screening, utilizing a rapid test or EIA format. Then, all positive patients would either be treated presumptively because the serious consequences of untreated infection far outweigh the effect of overtreatment, or have a follow-up RPR or VDRL to determine, if they have active infection before treatment. Treponemal tests are also used as diagnostic tests in patients with nonreactive nontreponemal tests, but with signs and symptoms of late syphilis. Treponemal tests are technically more difficult to perform and more expensive than nontreponemal tests. As with nontreponemal tests, false-positive reactions can occur with treponemal tests. Nevertheless, in the absence of immunosuppression, a nonreactive treponemal test is indicative of no past or present infection. There are many treponemal tests currently available, and some of the most commonly used treponemal tests are listed below.

Fluorescent treponemal antibody absorption test and fluorescent treponemal antibody absorption double staining tests: The fluorescent treponemal antibody absorption (FTA-ABS) test is an indirect fluorescent-antibody technique. In this procedure, serum samples are pretreated with an absorbent to remove nonspecific antibodies. The FTA-ABS double-staining test is a modification of the FTA-ABS test using a double-staining procedure with the addition of a contrasting counterstain. While these tests are highly sensitive and specific, they may produce variable results due to variation in equipment, reagents, and interpretation.

Treponema pallidum particle agglutination test: The *T. pallidum* particle agglutination (TP-PA) test is a qualitative assay for the detection of antibodies to *T. pallidum* in serum or plasma. This test is based on the agglutination of colored particle carriers sensitized with *T. pallidum* antigen and has replaced its predecessor, the microhemagglutination assay for *T. pallidum* (MHA-TP). The TP-PA test uses the same treponemal antigen as the MHA-TP test, but offers the advantage of gelatin particles instead of erythrocytes, thus, eliminating nonspecific reactions with plasma samples. The TP-PA test is less expensive and less complicated than the FTA-ABS tests, and the results are read with the unaided eye. It is one of the more commonly used treponemal tests. A positive TP-PA test in conjunction with a positive nontreponemal test is indicative of current or past infection with *T. pallidum.* The TP-PA test found to be an appropriate substitute for the MHA-TP test is as sensitive as the FTA-ABS test in primary syphilis and as useful as the RPR test in monitoring therapy.

Western blot: This is similar to the western blot test used for the confirmation of HIV antibodies, and provides a molecular characterization of the antibody response through the visualization of characteristic banding patterns. Western blot methods using whole cell lysate and recombinant antigens have been developed. Antibody reactivity to some of the treponemal antigenic bands is highly specific for syphilis. This test can detect either IgG or IgM antibodies and is considered a very useful adjunct confirmatory test.

Rapid tests: Treponemal tests are also commercially available in formats that can be performed at the point of care. They are available either as agglutination tests using latex particles coated with treponemal antigen or as immunochromatographic strips on which a positive reaction appears as a colored line. Most of these tests can be used with whole blood, serum or plasma. They can be stored at room temperature, are simple to perform, require minimal training and no equipment, and the results can be read visually in less than 30 minutes. Because rapid tests do not contain internal quality control, periodic external quality control using laboratory-based tests is recommended.

False-positive and False-negative Serological Reactions

The phospholipid antibodies detected by nontreponemal tests are not only produced in syphilis and other treponemal disease, but also in response to a variety of conditions unrelated to syphilis. Therefore, false-positive nontreponemal test reactions can have multiple causes. Their incidence is generally 1–2%. The rate of false-positives during pregnancy is no greater than that seen in the general population, but is higher among intravenous drug users. Generally, up to 90% of false-positive reactions have a titre of less than 1:8, and reactive nontreponemal tests with titres less than 1:8, and subsequent nonreactive treponemal tests are considered to be biological false-positive reactions. Chronic false-positive reactions persist for more than 6 months and are often associated with autoimmune disorders and chronic inflammatory conditions. False-positive reactions can also occur with treponemal tests, but this is less common than with nontreponemal tests.

Both types of tests can also yield false-negative results due to the prozone phenomenon. Such false-negatives occur in 1–2% of patients, especially in pregnant women and HIV patients. Serum from such patients should be tested at a 1:16 dilution. This, however, requires that the laboratory is given the relevant information from the patient's history and clinical diagnosis.

Evaluation of Treatment Efficacy

Definite criteria for treatment success or failure have not been established, and assessing response to treatment is often difficult. Also, treatment failure cannot be reliably distinguished from reinfection. Generally, the efficacy of therapy is monitored by a remission of symptoms and a decline in antibody titre as measured by nontreponemal tests. Sequential antibody titres should be measured using the same test in the same laboratory. A post-treatment fall in titre confirms response to treatment, and a rise in titre indicates treatment failure or reinfection. Typically, the phospholipid antibody titre declines by fourfold after 3 months (e.g., from 1:32 to 1:8) and by eightfold after 6 months (e.g., from 1:32 to 1:4) with standard therapy. However, there is evidence that 15% of treated patients with early syphilis will not show a fourfold decline in titre at 1 year post-treatment. The time for decline in antibody titre may be longer with the RPR test than with the VDRL test. HIV co-infection may delay the decline in titre, both in primary and secondary syphilis. CDC guidelines suggest that failure to achieve a fourfold decline in antibody titre by 6 months after therapy for primary and secondary syphilis and within 12–24 months in latent syphilis with initial high titres identifies patients at risk for treatment failure. Seroreversion is a slow process that depends on the stage of the disease and a number of other conditions. Therefore, the rate of decline in titre is more useful than seroreversion. To follow seroreversion, serum must be examined every 3–6 months for at least 2 years. After successful treatment, the RPR and VDRL tests usually become nonreactive after 1 year in patients with primary syphilis, after 2 years in patients with

Genital Dermatoses

secondary syphilis, and after 5 years in latent syphilis. Regardless, in some patients, particularly those treated in the latent or late stages, nontreponemal antibodies can persist at a low titre for a long period of time, sometimes for life, and this is referred to as the "serofast reaction". On the other hand, even without treatment, a patient may become serologically negative after several years. The VDRL test may be negative in up to one fourth of patients with untreated late syphilis. Treponemal antibody titres correlate poorly with disease activity and should not be used to monitor treatment. PCR may be useful to rule out persistent infection. However, IgM-specific treponemal tests may be useful for monitoring treatment status and response to therapy. Nevertheless, untreated and inadequately treated infections beyond early stages, as well as reinfections, cannot be excluded based on a negative IgM test.

Treatment

All persons with syphilis should be counseled concerning the risks of HIV infection and other STIs and testing for these infections should be offered.

- *Early syphilis*: (Primary, secondary, or latent syphilis of not more than two years duration)
  - Recommended regimen: Benzathine benzylpenicillin, 2.4 million IU by intramuscular injection, at a single session. Because of the volume involved, this dose is usually given as two injections at separate sites.
  - Alternative regimen: Procaine benzylpenicillin, 1.2 million IU by intramuscular injection, daily for 10 consecutive days.
    - Alternative regimen for penicillin-allergic nonpregnant patients: Doxycycline, 100 mg orally, twice daily for 14 days or tetracycline, 500 mg orally, 4 times daily for 14 days
    - Alternative regimen for penicillin-allergic pregnant patients: Erythromycin, 500 mg orally, 4 times daily for 14 days.
- *Late latent syphilis:* (Infection of more than two years duration without evidence of treponemal infection)

- Recommended regimen: Benzathine benzylpenicillin, 2.4 million IU by intramuscular injection, once weekly for 3 consecutive weeks
- Alternative regimen: Procaine benzylpenicillin, 1.2 million IU by intramuscular injection, once daily for 20 consecutive days.
  - Alternative regimen for penicillin-allergic nonpregnant patients: Doxycycline, 100 mg orally, twice daily for 30 days or tetracycline, 500 mg orally, four times daily for 30 days
  - Alternative regimen for penicillin-allergic pregnant patients: Erythromycin 500 mg orally, four times daily for 30 days.
- *Neurosyphilis*
  - Recommended regimen: Aqueous benzylpenicillin 12-24 million IU by intravenous injection, administered daily in doses of 2-4 million IU, every 4 hours for 14 days.
  - Alternative regimen: Procaine benzylpenicillin, 1.2 million IU by intramuscular injection, once daily, and probenecid, 500 mg orally, four times daily, both for 10-14 days.
    - Alternative regimen for penicillin-allergic nonpregnant patients: Doxycycline, 200 mg orally, twice daily for 30 days or tetracycline, 500 mg orally, four times daily for 30 days.
- *Congenital syphilis:*
  - Early congenital syphilis (up to 2 years of age) and infants with abnormal CSF:
    - Recommended regimen: Aqueous benzylpenicillin 100,000-150,000 IU/kg/day administered as 50,000 IU/kg/dose IV every 12 hours, during the first 7 days of life and every 8 hours thereafter for a total of 10 days or procaine benzylpenicillin, 50,000 IU/kg by intramuscular injection, as a single daily dose for 10 days.
  - Congenital syphilis of two or more years:
    - Recommended regimen: Aqueous benzylpenicillin, 200,000-300,000 IU/kg/day by intravenous or intra-

muscular injection, administered as 50,000 IU/kg/dose every 4–6 hours for 10–14 days
- Alternative regimen for penicillin-allergic patients, after the first month of life: Erythromycin, 7.5–12.5 mg/kg orally, 4 times daily for 30 days.

SYNDROMIC MANAGEMENT

Genital ulcer disease (GUD) can have multifactorial causes. In regions where there are no diagnostic facilities or where the costs of diagnostic tests are prohibitive, syndromic management of GUD to cover common causes, such as chancroid and syphilis is recommended. If there is a history of genital blisters suggestive of genital herpes or in a region endemic for LGV or donovanosis, treatment should also cover for these organisms. This usually consists of a single dose of benzathine penicillin for syphilis, and a single dose of ciprofloxacin for chancroid. Syndromic algorithms for GUD were most effective in identifying syphilis and chancroid. Adding a RPR test to the algorithm for better detection of syphilis may disadvantage chancroid management. A positive RPR test may lead to treatment of syphilis only, and treatment for chancroid is missed in patients with dual infection. It is recommended that patients with a positive RPR should also be treated for chancroid. It is recommended that azithromycin 1 g or erythromycin 500 mg four times daily for 7 days be included to cover nongonococcal urethritis caused by *Chlamydia trachomatis* and *Mycoplasma genitalium*. The protocol for syndromic management should be modified accordingly as determined by the main causes of genital ulcers and concomitant STDs in each country. One of the major challenges is partner notification and provision of epidemiological treatment to sexual partners, otherwise public health control will fail. Syndromic case management protocol using the colour kits is given in Table 2.

GENITAL WART

Genital warts (or condylomata acuminata, venereal warts, anal warts, and anogenital warts) are symptoms of a highly contagious

TABLE 2: Syndromic case management protocol

Kit No.	Syndrome	Colour	Contents
Kit 1	Urethral discharge (UD), Cervical discharge (CD), Ano-rectal discharge (ARD), Painful scrotal swelling (PSS), Presumptive treatment (PT)	Grey	Tablet azithromycin 1 g (1) and Tablet cefixime 400 mg (1)
Kit 2	Vaginal discharge (VD)	Green	Tablet secnidazole 2 g (1) and Tablet fluconazol 150 mg (1)
Kit 3	Genital ulcer disease- non herpetic (GUD-NH)	White	Injection benzathin penicillin 2.4 MU (1) and Tablet azithromycin 1g (1) and disposable syringe 10 ml with 21 gauge needle (1) and sterile water 10 ml (1)
Kit 4	Genital ulcer disease-non herpetic (GUD-NH)–for patients allergic to penicillin	Blue	Tablet doxycycline 100 mg (30) and Tablet azithromycin 1 g (1)
Kit 5	Genital ulcer disease-herpetic (GUD-H)	Red	Tablet acyclovir 400 mg (21)
Kit 6	Lower abdominal pain (LAP/PID)	Yellow	Tablet cefixime 400 mg (1) and Tablet metroniadazole 400 mg (28) and Capsule doxycyclin 100 mg (28)
Kit 7	Inguinal bubo (IB)	Black	Tablet doxycyclin 100 mg (42) and Tablet azithromycin 1 g (1)

STD caused by some types of human papillomavirus (HPV). HPV is a group of nonenveloped, double-stranded DNA viruses belonging to the family papovaviridae. Viral replication is restricted to the basal cell layer of surface tissues. The virus will penetrate both the cutaneous and mucosal epithelium in search of the appropriate cellular host. It will subsequently invade and infect the basal keratinocytes of the epidermis. The mucosa can be infected anywhere along the genital tract, including the vulva, vagina, cervix, and perianal regions in females as well as the penile shaft, scrotum, periurethral, and perianal regions in males. Infected regions will be marked by a proliferation of viral DNA and the formation of a warty papule or plaque. The viral genome is composed of six early-open reading frames (E1, E2, E4, E5, E6, E7) and two late-open reading frames (L1, L2). The early-open E genes are important for regulatory function and encode proteins involved in viral replication and cell transformation. In contrast, the late-open L genes encode viral capsid proteins. Differences in the L1 genotype lead to slightly altered patterns of viral DNA replication, which are thought to account for the various HPV subtypes. Specifically, low-risk HPV subtypes will remain separate from the host cell DNA and thus undergo replication independently. In contrast, high-risk HPV subtypes will incorporate their DNA directly into the host cell's genetic material. The integration of viral and host cell DNA often results in the dysregulation and uncontrolled activation of the E6 and E7 genes, which promotes the transcription of oncoproteins. These will bind and inactivate tumor suppressor genes p53 and Rb, leading to increased cell proliferation and a greater risk of malignant progression.

More than 100 types of HPV exist, more than 40 of which can infect the genital area. Most HPV infections are asymptomatic, unrecognized, or subclinical. Oncogenic or high-risk HPV types (e.g., HPV types 16 and 18) are the cause of cervical cancers. These HPV types are also associated with other anogenital cancers in men and women, including penile, vulvar, vaginal, and anal cancer, as well a subset of oropharyngeal cancers. Nononcogenic or low-risk HPV types (e.g., HPV types 6 and 11), are the cause of genital warts and recurrent respiratory papillomatosis. Persistent oncogenic HPV infection is the strongest risk factor for development of precancers and cancers.

Human papillomavirus 2, 4, 7, 26, 27, 28, and 29 commonly cause warts on the skin (most often on the hands, feet, knuckles, and periungual areas). Lesions of the respiratory tract or respiratory papillomatosis are most commonly caused by HPV 6 and 11, acquired by vertical transmission in the perinatal period or by sexual transmission. One-third to one-half of children born to mothers with HPV genital infection are positive for HPV DNA by oral and respiratory swabs; however, only 1/400 children is at risk for respiratory papillomatosis. HPV can also cause papillomas in the oral cavity and in the conjunctiva.

It is spread through direct skin-to-skin contact usually during oral, genital, or anal sex with an infected partner. Rarely, genital HPV infection with low-risk types is transmitted from mother to newborn during delivery and can cause respiratory tract warts in the child known as juvenile-onset recurrent respiratory papillomatosis.

Risk factors consistently associated with genital HPV infection:
- Young age
- Increasing number of recent and lifetime sex partners
- Early age of first sexual intercourse
- Sexual behavior of sex partners
- Multiple sex partners
- Lack of circumcision in men.

Genital HPV infects the basal cell layer of stratified squamous epithelium and stimulates cellular proliferation. Affected cells display a broad spectrum of changes, ranging from benign hyperplasia, to dysplasia, to invasive carcinoma. The lesions appear after an incubation period of 1–8 months, with an average of 3 months.

Clinical manifestations of genital HPV infection include:
- Genital warts
- Cervical cellular abnormalities detected by Pap tests
- Anogenital squamous cell cancers, oropharyngeal cancers, and
- Recurrent respiratory papillomatosis.

Genital warts have five morphologic types:
1. Smooth papules: Usually dome-shaped and skin-colored
2. Flat papules: Macular to slightly raised, flesh-colored with smooth surface. More commonly found on internal structures (i.e., cervix), but also occur on external genitalia
3. Keratotic warts: Thick horny layer resembling common warts or seborrheic keratosis
4. Giant condyloma (Buschke-Lowenstein tumor): This is a very rare variant of HPV 6 and 11-associated disease, characterized by aggressive downgrowth into the underlying dermal structures

Genital Dermatoses

5. Condylomata acuminata: Cauliflower-like appearance, skin-colored, pink or hyperpigmented. May be keratotic on skin; generally nonkeratinized on mucosal surfaces.

Genital warts appear most commonly in areas of coital friction (Figs 10 to 19).
- Men—penis, scrotum, urethral meatus, and perianal area
- Women—introitus, vulva, perineum, and perianal area.

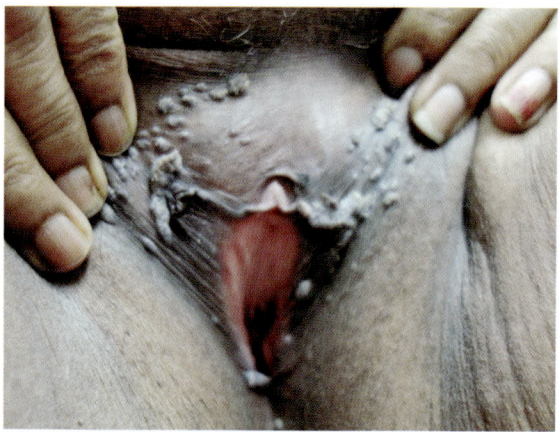

Figure 10: Genital wart in a sex worker

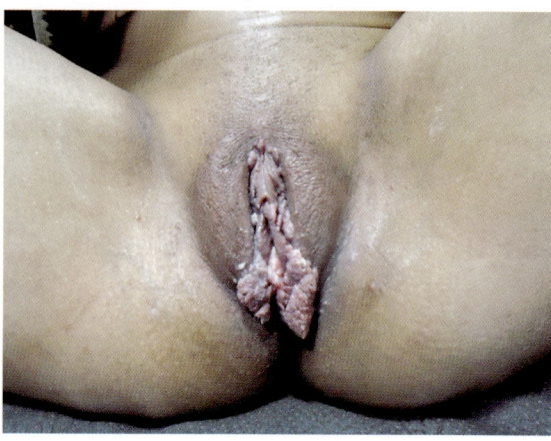

Figure 11: Genital wart in a pregnant woman

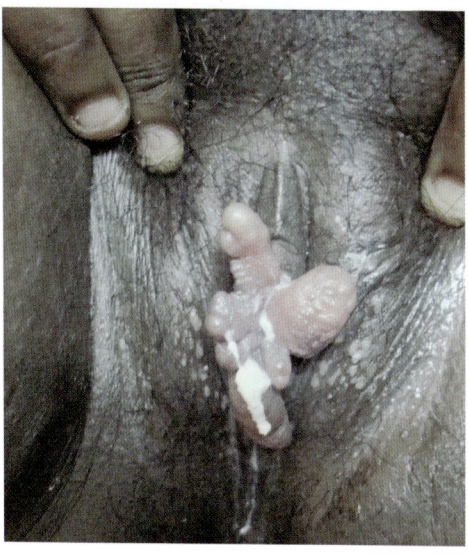

Figure 12: Genital wart in a human immunodeficiency virus positive pregnant woman with mucosal edema, candidiasis. Note the subungual wart

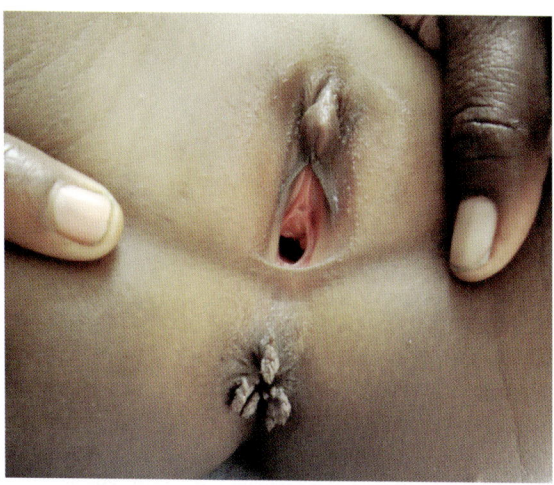

Figure 13: Perianal wart in a girl following child abuse

Genital Dermatoses

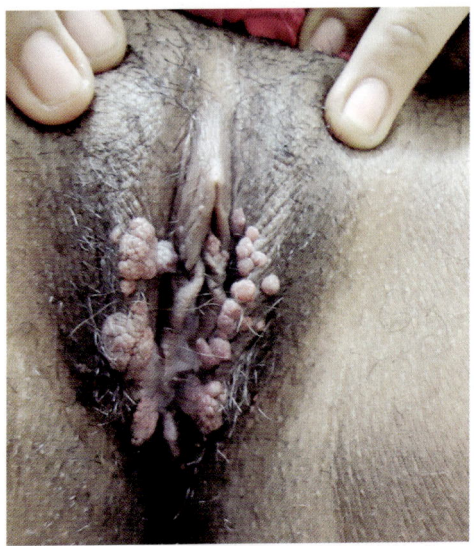

Figure 14: Multiple warts recalcitrant to treatment in HIV positive woman

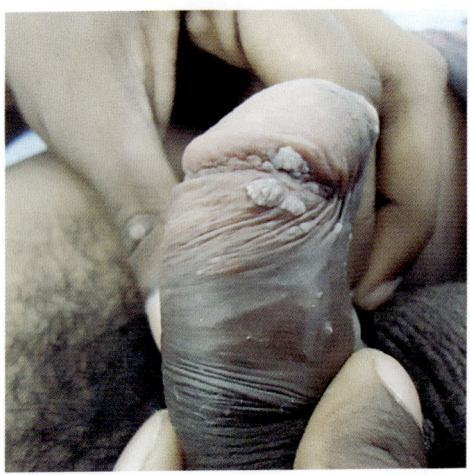

Figure 15: Penile genital wart, verrucous papules over coronal sulcus and glans

Sexually Transmitted Infection Affecting the Genitalia

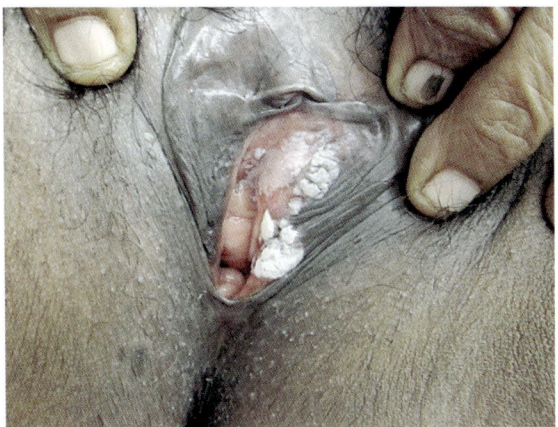

Figure 16: Genital wart over labial skin and mucosa in a diabetic woman

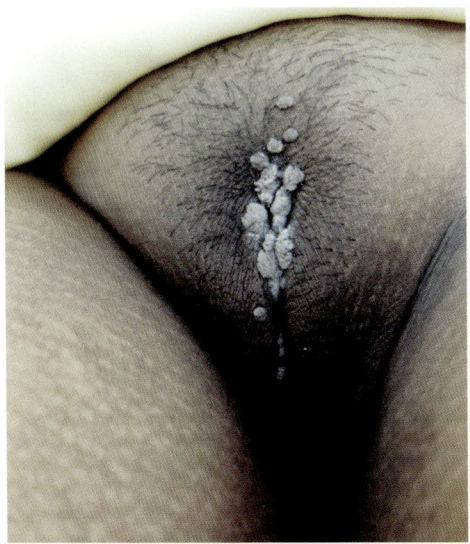

Figure 17: Genital wart in an adolescent girl

Genital Dermatoses

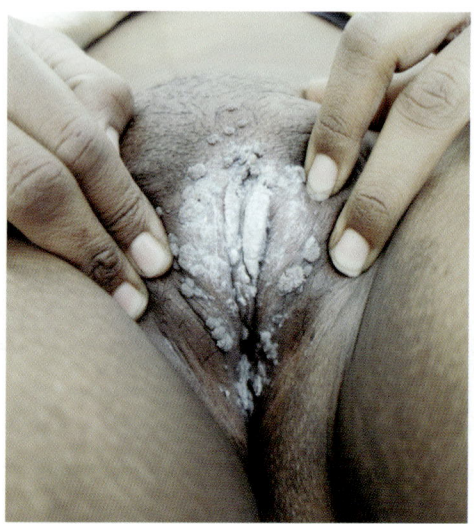

Figure 18: Same girl as in Fig 17

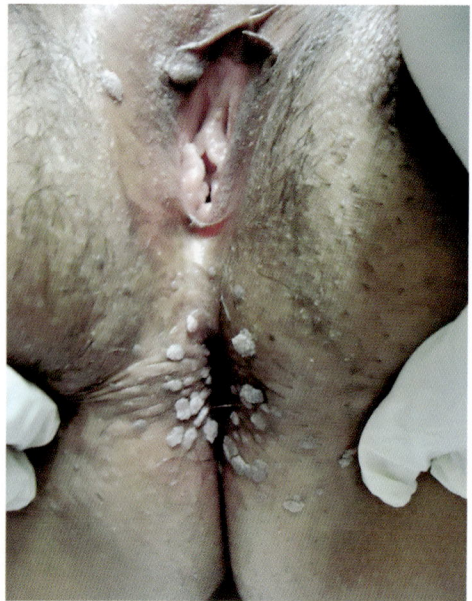

Figure 19: Genital and perianal wart

Less common sites:
- Cervix and vaginal walls in women
- Pubic area, upper thighs, or crural folds in men and women.

Perianal warts do not necessarily imply anal intercourse, but may be secondary to autoinoculation, sexual activity other than intercourse or spread from a nearby genital wart site. Intra-anal warts are seen predominantly in patients who have had receptive anal intercourse.

Anogenital warts in children have serious medical, social, and legal implications. Concerns including possible sexual abuse, vertical transmission from the mother, and the potential for the future development of anogenital malignancies in children with anogenital warts must be addressed.

Symptoms

- Genital warts usually cause no symptoms
- Vulvar warts can cause dyspareunia, pruritis, and burning discomfort
- Penile warts occasionally cause pruritis
- Urethral meatal warts occasionally cause hematuria or impairment of urinary stream
- Vaginal warts occasionally cause discharge, bleeding or obstruction of birth canal (due to increased wart growth in pregnancy)
- Perianal and intra-anal warts occasionally cause pain, bleeding on defecation or pruritis
- Anogenital warts in chidren can be the result of child abuse.

Cervical Cancer and Human Papillomavirus

An estimated 493,000 new cases of cervical cancer were recognized in 2002, along with approximately 274,000 deaths from cervical cancer in the same year. Of these cases, 80% occur in developing countries. In India, the annual incidence is approximately 130,000 new cases, with 70,000–75,000 deaths annually; India carries greater than 25% of the global burden of cervical cancer-related deaths. HPV

Genital Dermatoses

infection is considered a necessary condition for the development of cancer. The majority of cases are squamous cell carcinomas (SCCs), while adenocarcinomas are less common. Globally, HPV 16 is most prevalent in SCCs, while HPV 18 is most prevalent in adenocarcinomas; together, HPV 16 and 18 account for 70% of cervical cancers. In India, however, HPV 16 is the most prevalent type in both SCCs and adenocarcinomas, accounting for approximately 90% of all cervical cancers. As cervical cancer affects women at a relatively younger age than other cancers, the years of life lost (YLL) worldwide in 2000 was estimated to be 2.7 million; cervical cancer is the largest single cause of YLL from cancer in the developing world.

Complications of Untreated Human Papillomavirus Infection

Both low-risk (subtypes 6 and 11) and high-risk (subtypes 16 and 18) HPV subtypes have also been associated with the very low-grade, well-differentiated SCC known as verrucous carcinoma (VC). VC is divided into clinicopathological types based on the anatomic area of involvement: oral florid papillomatosis (oral cavity), giant condyloma of Buschke and Lowenstein (anogenital area), and carcinoma cuniculatum (palmoplantar surface). These tumors tend to spread by local invasion and therefore, rarely metastasize. While a direct causal relationship between HPV and VC has yet to be defined, it is hypothesized that HPV's viral oncogene expression promotes the degradation of the p53 tumor suppression gene, thereby lowering the threshold for tumor formation. Histologically, VC can vary from benign-appearing pseudoepitheliomatous hyperplasia-like lesions to invasive SCC. Additionally, presence of vacuolation and prominent keratohyalin granules in the stratum granulosa cells, which are hallmark features of genital warts, was discovered to be variable in histological studies of VC. One can differentiate VC and SCC by comparing the immunoperoxidase staining pattern of expression of certain oncogenes. For instance, VC and SCC cells can stain positively for bcl-2, Ki-67, and p53. However, nuclei of VC stain positive for p53 and Ki-67 in the lower third of the epidermis, primarily in the basal proliferating cells. The nuclei of SCC stain positive throughout the full thickness of the epidermis for these markers.

Additionally, while most HPV infections clear spontaneously, in 10-20% of women these infections persist and these females are at risk for progression to grade two third cervical intraepithelial neoplasm and, if left untreated, can eventually develop invasive cancer of the cervix. Penile cancer, which is ten times less common than cervical cancer, also has a high correlation rate with high-risk HPV infection.

Diagnosis

Diagnosis is usually made by visual inspection with bright light. Usually the diagnosis is made clinically. Biopsy is seldom necessary to accurately diagnose visible genital warts.

The histological characteristics of the classical protuberant growth type of condyloma acuminatum are as follows:
- Hyperkeratosis and parakeratosis of varying degree
- Moderate granulomatosis
- Acanthosis and papillomatosis
- Mitotic figures may be present in the epidermis
- The most characteristic feature is the presence of "koilocytes", which are mature squamous cells with a large, clear perinuclear zone and smudgy nuclei, scattered through the outer cell layers.

Mild acetic acid soaking should not be used routinely to screen patients.

Cytology (Pap test) is a useful screening test to detect cervical dysplasia (not HPV per se). It provides indirect evidence of HPV, because it detects squamous epithelial cell changes that are almost always due to HPV.

Colposcopy, meatoscopy, and proctoscopy for detecting cervical, meatal, and anal warts, respectively.

Southern blot hybridization technique is the gold standard among HPV DNA detection methods, but is too time consuming and labor intensive for routine diagnosis.

Genital Dermatoses

In situ hybridization helps in determining the localization of HPV DNA within the specimen.

Polymerase chain reaction is the most sensitive method for detection of HPV DNA, being able to detect one viral genome in 100,000 cells.

Differential Diagnosis

- Condylomata lata of secondary syphilis
- Molluscum contagiosum
- Seborrheic keratosis
- Lichen planus
- Psoriasis
- Melanocytic nevus
- Pink pearly penile papules
- Squamous cell carcinoma in situ
- Bowenoid papulosis.

Treatment

Treatment options are classified as follows:
- Home therapy: Podophyllotoxin (0.5% solution or 0.15% cream) and imiquimod
- Hospital therapy: Electrosurgery, laser ablation, curettage, cryotherapy, trichloroacetic acid, and podophyllin
- Therapies not generally recommended: Used only in special situations, these include interferons and 5-fluorouracil.

Podophyllotoxin 0.05% Solution or Gel and 0.15% Cream (Podofilox)

Podophyllotoxin is a purified extract of the podophyllum plant, which binds to cellular microtubules, inhibits mitotic division, and induces necrosis of warts that is maximal 3–5 days after administration. Shallow erosions occur as the lesions necrotize and heal within a few days to weeks. Typically, the solution is recommended for penile lesions, whereas cream or gel vehicle preparations are thought to be more comfortable for application to anal or vaginal lesions. This treatment option is generally thought to be safe, effective, and can be self-administered. Podophyllotoxin is available as a solution, cream or gel and must be applied twice daily for three consecutive days of the week, for a maximum of four patients should apply podofilox solution with a cotton swab, or finger, to visible genital warts twice a day for 3 days, followed by 4 days of no therapy. This cycle may be repeated as necessary for up to four cycles. Total wart area treated should not exceed 10 cm^2, and a total volume of podofilox should be limited to 0.5 mL per day.

Imiquimod 5% Cream

Imiquimod (imidazoquinolinamine) 5% cream is a patient-applied topical immunomodulatory agent, which first received its indication for the treatment of external CA in 1997. It has since been used in the treatment of a variety of skin conditions, including basal cell carcinomas and actinic keratosis. Although its precise mechanism of action remains unclear, imiquimod is believed to activate immune cells by binding to the membranous toll-like receptor. This leads to the secretion of multiple cytokines, such as interferon-α, interleukin-6, and tumor necrosis factor-α, which are critical in the induction of an inflammatory response promoting wart clearance. In addition, imiquimod-treated patients have been shown to have a decrease in viral load measured by HPV DNA, a decrease in messenger ribonucleic acid (mRNA) expression for markers of keratinocyte proliferation, and an increase in mRNA expression for markers of tumor suppression.

Patients should apply imiquimod cream once daily at bedtime, three times a week for up to 16 weeks. The treatment area should be washed with soap and water 6–10 hours after the application. Commonly encountered local inflammatory side effects, such as itching, erythema, burning, irritation, tenderness, ulceration, and pain have been long-standing issues with the 5% cream. Occasionally, patients may experience systemic side effects of headaches, muscle aches, fatigue, and general malaise.

Podophyllin

Podophyllin is a resinous mixture extracted from the dried rhizome and roots of *Podophyllum emodi* (found in the Himalayan regions of northern India) and *Podophyllum peltatum* (Mayapple or American mandrake found in North America). The resin content of *P. emodi* (6-12%) is approximately twice that of *P. peltatum* (2-8%). Apply topically as a solution containing 10-25% podophyllum resin in benzoin tincture, sparingly to intact HPV warts and allow to air dry. Adjacent skin may be protected by applying petrolatum or flexible collodion prior to application of the drug. The preparation area should be thoroughly washed off 1-4 hours after application to reduce local irritation. The procedure can be repeated once a week. After six sittings, if the wart persists, other treatment modalities need to be considered.

Trichloroacetic Acid

Treatment via chemical cautery with a solution of 60-90% trichloroacetic acid (TCA) is most effective when treating few small, moist lesions, although TCA also can be used for vaginal or anal lesions. A small amount should be applied and allowed to dry until a white frosting develops. Successful treatment of warts can occasionally occur with as little as a single dose; however, more frequently, several applications are required. Additionally, the low danger of systemic absorption allows for safe application during pregnancy. The main side effects of acid treatments involve pain or burning during administration as well as destruction of the healthy tissue surrounding the wart. The latter can be minimized by washings with soap and sodium bicarbonate immediately following over-application, and dermal injury or scarring is rare.

Sinecatechins 15% Ointment (Grade A)

Sinecatechins is a botanical extract approved in 2006 by the United States FDA for the treatment of genital warts, making it the first botanical to officially receive medical approval. The active ingredient is a green tea extract containing sinecatechins, which is thought to possess antioxidant, antiviral, and antitumor effects. Although the precise mechanism of action remains unclear, sinecatechins is thought to modulate the inflammatory response through the inhibition of transcription factors activator protein 1 (AP-1) and nuclear factor kappa-light-chain-enhancer of activated B cells (NF-κB), both of which are induced by reactive oxygen species. They have also been shown to downregulate the expression of cyclooxygenase-2, which has been linked to activation of the prostaglandin E2 system and subsequent epithelial dysplasia.

Sinecatechins 15% cream is applied topically to warts three times a day for up to 4 months. Typically, if an improvement is not seen within a few weeks, the treatment is stopped and another option is tried. This botanical extract is associated with a number of adverse effects that are thought to occur in approximately 20% of users. These events are generally quite mild and typically include redness, burning, itching, and pain at the site of application. More severe reactions associated with this topical product's use, such as lymphadenitis, vulvovaginitis, balanitis, and ulceration are extremely rare, but have been reported.

Cryotherapy

Cryotherapy is a process in which the abnormal tissue is frozen through the use of a cooling agent, such as nitrous oxide or liquid nitrogen. Temperatures must be exorbitantly cold so as to cause permanent dermal and vascular damage. This leads to the initiation of an immune repair response, resulting in the necrosis and clearance of the destroyed cells. Generally, this treatment is most effective when used for multiple small warts on the penile shaft or vulva.

Cryotherapy is considered a fairly inexpensive and highly successful therapy, with a 79–88% clearance rate seen within the first three treatments. This suggests a more efficacious outcome when compared with TCA. Cryotherapy has various limiting factors. Variables in administration, such as the temperature utilized and time of contact, influence efficacy of treatment. Common side effects of cryotherapy include local tissue destruction, such as painful blistering, ulceration, infection, potentially permanent scarring, and loss of pigmentation, which can be slightly more severe than that of TCA. Other disadvantages of cryotherapy are that multiple outpatient visits are required and the pain associated with its application can limit its repeated use in certain subjects. However, the effects of cryotherapy are entirely local, making it the current therapy of choice for pregnant women with multiple warts.

Electrosurgery (Grade B)

Electrosurgery involves the use of high-frequency electrical currents in the form of thermal coagulation or electrocautery to burn and destroy warty lesions. The desiccated tissue is subsequently removed by curettage. This technique is particularly efficacious when used in the treatment of smaller warts located on the shaft of the penis, the rectum, or the vulva; however, it is not recommended for large lesions as it may lead to permanent scar formation. Electrosurgery is an extremely effective technique with randomized controlled trials yielding clearance rates as high as 94% measured 6 weeks post-treatment. These rates, however, tend to normalize after 3 months, suggesting that electrosurgery is comparable to cryotherapy with regard to it's long-term effectiveness. Electrosurgery is also a fairly painful procedure and local or general anesthesia is usually required. Side effects tend to be relatively minimal and are typically limited to postprocedural pain, although the use of general anesthesia is always associated with a certain degree of elevated risk. It is important to note that electrosurgery is contraindicated in patients with cardiac pacemakers or other implanted cardiac devices due to the potentially fatal effects of current interference and the disruption of the pacemaker rhythms.

Surgical Scissor Excision (Grade B)

One of the oldest documented treatments for the removal of genital warts, surgical excision was considered for many years to be the primary available option. It involves the physical removal of diseased tissue from the body with scissors or a scalpel, followed by suturing the remaining healthy skin together. It is associated with up to a 72% clearance rate, which is evident immediately and often persisting over a year later. Although now considered to be somewhat outdated, this treatment option is still suitable for very large lesions that may be causing obstruction and are ineligible or unresponsive to other forms of treatment. Examples include lesions involving the urethral meatus. Additionally, surgical excision remains the optimal procedure for the removal of neoplastic lesions suspected of malignant progression, which must be submitted for further histopathological examination. Surgical removal of large lesions is a painful process, which frequently results in bleeding and scar formation. The administration of local or general anesthesia is commonly recommended.

Carbon dioxide Laser Therapy (Grade B)

Carbon dioxide (CO_2) laser therapy relies upon the use of a concentrated beam of infrared light energy, which will heat and eventually vaporize the targeted areas. The intense light energy has the added benefit of providing immediate cauterization of any ligated vessels, ensuring a virtually bloodless procedure. The spatial confinement of the laser beam permits precise tissue ablation resulting in rapid healing with little or no scar formation. The efficacy of CO_2 therapy for CA remains contentious. Laser therapy is typically considered to be less effective than other forms of surgical treatment, with clearance rates ranging between 23 and 52%. Recurrence rates also tend to be elevated, reaching as high as 77%. Side effects are generally mild and limited to the burning of tissue surrounding the lesion. Despite these seemingly unfavorable results, the deep penetrating effect of the laser often allows for a greater and more complete viral attack than seen with other surgical treatment options. This renders it the treatment of choice for immunosuppressed individuals as well as for pregnant women with extensive lesions who remain unresponsive to TCA or cryotherapy.

Therapies Not Generally Recommended

5-fluorouracil and interferon therapy are not recommended for use in the primary care setting. 5-fluorouracil is one of the oldest chemotherapeutic agents and has been effectively used in the treatment of cancer for more than 40 years. Although not officially approved by the FDA for use in the treatment of genital warts, topical 5-fluorouracil is still seen as a favorable option for urethral warts. The administration of 5-fluorouracil has historically been associated with highly variable response rates, and side effects tend to be slightly more severe than those of imiquimod 5% cream with comparable clearance rates yet marginally higher rates of recurrence.

Historically, interferon therapy has been used predominantly for the treatment of malignant melanoma; however, recent evidence suggests that it may be useful as either an individual or adjuvant to surgical treatment of genital warts. Interferon therapy can be administered systemically, via oral or intramuscular injection, as well as locally, via direct intralesional injections. Typically, 1–1.5 million units is used, and injections occur three times a week for duration of 3 weeks. The use of interferon therapy for the treatment of genital warts remains somewhat controversial.

Management in Pregnancy

Genital warts can proliferate and become more friable during pregnancy.
- Cytotoxic agents (podophyllin, podofilox, imiquimod) should not be used
- Cryotherapy, TCA, and surgical removal may be used.

Patients with suppressed cell immunity associated with organ transplantation, HIV infection or other conditions may have a poorer response to treatment for genital warts, increased relapse rates, and a higher risk of dysplasia.

Human Papillomavirus Vaccines

- The bivalent vaccine (HPV2), Cervarix, protects against two HPV types (16 and 18), which are responsible for 70% of cervical cancers
- The quadrivalent vaccine (HPV4), Gardasil, protects against four HPV types (6, 11, 16, and 18), which are responsible for 70% of cervical cancers (16 and 18) and 90% of genital warts (6 and 11).

Ideally, the vaccines should be administered before onset of sexual activity. However, persons who are sexually active also may benefit from vaccination.

A prophylactic vaccine against HPV infection is currently approved for use in India. Gardasil is a quadrivalent vaccine, effective against HPV types 6, 11, 16, and 18, the major types causing anogenital warts as well as cervical cancer. The vaccine utilizes the major capsid protein L1 of specific HPV types, which has the ability to self-assemble into virus-like particles. Infection is prevented through the induction of neutralizing antibodies against L1. Gardasil is currently dosed in a series of three intramuscular injections.

Although a bivalent vaccine that protects against HPV types 16 and 18 is available, Cervarix, it has not yet been approved for use in India. Both vaccines provide protection against cervical cancer, but the added protection of the quadrivalent vaccine against the HPV types that cause the majority of anogenital warts is of particular importance to dermatologists. The advantage with this formulation is while some at-risk patients, both male and female, may not recognize the importance of vaccination against an internal malignancy without external manifestations; they are more likely to embrace a vaccine that can prevent visible anogenital warts and the associated stigma. Widespread vaccination against anogenital warts carries the additional benefit of protection against cervical cancer as well as likely protection against many other HPV-associated malignancies. In addition, there is a potential for partners of vaccinated males to receive the indirect benefit of decreased transmission of concomitant high-risk HPV types. By recommending HPV vaccination to their patients, dermatologists can directly impact the morbidity and mortality of anogenital warts and cervical cancer in India, in both vaccines and potentially, their partners.

Current American recommendations for the quadrivalent vaccination, given by the CDC and American Academy of Pediatrics (AAP), are routine vaccination of girls ages 11-12 (in most cases, prior to the onset of sexual activity) and catch-up vaccination of girls ages 13-26. Although women who are sexually active may have already been infected with HPV, vaccination confers protection against the remaining genotypes. The vaccine can be given to patients who have

Genital Dermatoses

abnormal or equivocal Pap smear results, who are breastfeeding or who are immunocompromised (both acquired and iatrogenic).

Several barriers exist to introduction of HPV vaccines for widespread use in India and other developing nations. Historically, inhabitants of developing nations have had to wait decades before new vaccines became available through their national immunization programs. Large-scale immunogenicity and efficacy trials must be conducted in these populations prior to approval for widespread use. Vaccination of adolescents, especially in three doses is more logistically difficult than vaccination of newborns. Social attitudes toward sexual behavior in India are more conservative than those of Western nations, and thus the acceptance of a vaccine for a STI is likely lower. Lack of education relating to vaccines and the fear that the vaccine may actually cause the disease it is intended to prevent may also decrease acceptance. The vaccine is relatively expensive, and long-term efficacy has yet to be proven, both of which are barriers to appropriation of resources for its inclusion in mass vaccination programs. In addition, the HPV vaccine must compete for already scarce resources against vaccines for other diseases that cause significant morbidity and mortality in childhood. Although, both the bivalent and quadrivalent vaccines protect against HPV 16, the most prevalent type in India, there is no vaccine that protects against all oncogenic HPV types. Thus, there will be a continued need for screening of vaccinated women, as there is no guarantee that they will not develop cervical cancer from another HPV types.

HERPES GENITALIS

Genital herpes is an infection caused by the herpes simplex virus (HSV) and is generally found on the genitals and nearby areas. There are two main types of HSV: type 1, which is mainly associated with facial infections and type 2, which is mainly genital, although there is considerable overlap. Clinically, about 60–70% of primary genital infections are due to herpes simplex virus 2 (HSV-2) with the rest due to HSV-1.

Sexually Transmitted Infection Affecting the Genitalia

Definitions

Primary infection: Recently acquired infection with HSV-1 or HSV-2 with an absence of antibodies to either type on serological testing.

Nonprimary infection: Recently acquired infection with a virus type in the presence of antibodies to the other virus type e.g., HSV-2 in a person with previous antibodies to HSV-1 but absence of antibodies to HSV-2 on serological testing.

First episode: The first clinical episode of genital HSV-1 or HSV-2. This may present as a primary HSV infection or a new nonprimary infection or a recurrence of a previously asymptomatic infection. It is not possible to reliably distinguish between these on clinical grounds alone.

Recurrence: Previously acquired HSV-1 or HSV-2 infection with antibodies to the same type on serological testing.

Pathophysiology

Both, type 1 and type 2 HSVs, reside in a latent state in the nerves that supply sensation to the skin. HSV invades and replicates in neurons as well as in epidermal and dermal cells. Virions travel from the initial site of infection on the skin or mucosa to the sensory dorsal root ganglion, where latency is established. Viral replication in the sensory ganglia leads to recurrent clinical outbreaks. These outbreaks can be induced by various stimuli, such as trauma, ultraviolet radiation, and extremes in temperature, stress, immunosuppression, or hormonal fluctuations. Viral shedding, leading to possible transmission, occurs during primary infection, during subsequent recurrences, and during periods of asymptomatic viral shedding.

Transmission

Direct skin-to-skin contact spreads HSV infection most easily. Thus, sexual contact, including orogenital contact, is the most common way to transmit genital HSV infection. The virus can be shed in saliva and genital secretions from individuals, even if they have no symptoms, especially in the days and weeks following a clinical episode. The amount shed during active lesions is 100 to 1000 times greater. Asymptomatic shedding is a common occurrence whether or not clinical signs of the disease are present. Minor injury helps spread the virus, especially into the skin. Vertical (mother to baby) transmission or auto (self) inoculation may also occur.

Clinical Features

Classic presentation:
- Painful vesiculopustular lesions
- Genital ulcers
- Perianal and anal ulcers.

Atypical Presentation:
- Genital itching
- Vulvar, scrotal, or perianal fissures
- Cervicitis or proctitis
- Urethral or vaginal discharge
- Vulvar or perianal irritation
- Dysuria
- Penile or scrotal irritation
- Painless ulcers.

Primary Infection

Primary herpes genitalis occurs within 2 days to 2 weeks after exposure to the virus and has the most severe clinical manifestations. Symptoms of the primary episode typically last for 2–3 weeks. In men, painful, erythematous, vesicular lesions that ulcerate most commonly occur on the penis, but they can also occur on the anus and the perineum. In women, primary herpes genitalis presents as vesicular or ulcerated lesions on the cervix and as painful vesicles on the external genitalia bilaterally. They can also occur on the vagina, the perineum, the buttocks, and at times, the legs in a sacral nerve distribution. Associated symptoms include fever, malaise, edema, inguinal lymphadenopathy, dysuria, and vaginal or penile discharge. It is not uncommon to see patients with both HSV-1 and HSV-2 infection at a given point of time (Figs 20 to 26). Females may also have lumbosacral radiculopathy, and as many as 25% of women with primary HSV-2 infections may have associated aseptic meningitis.

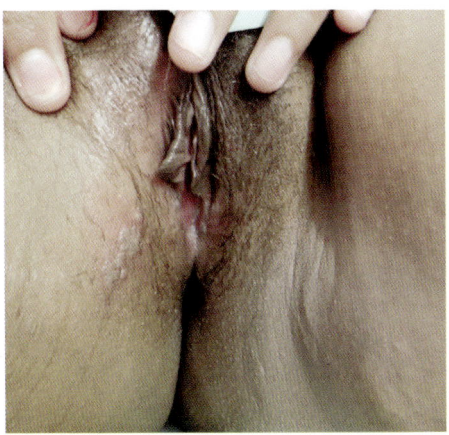

Figure 20: Herpes simplex early intact vesicles. Note the grouping and surrounding erythema

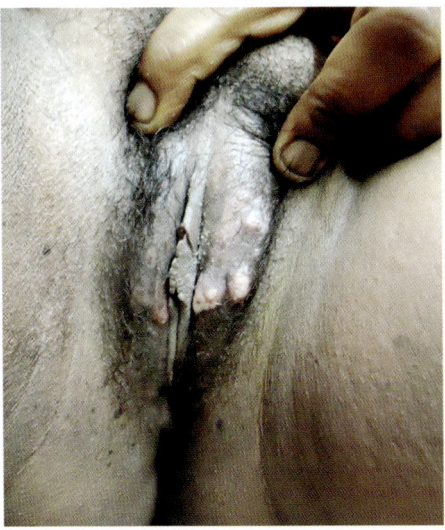

Figure 21: Genital herpes with secondary infection

Genital Dermatoses

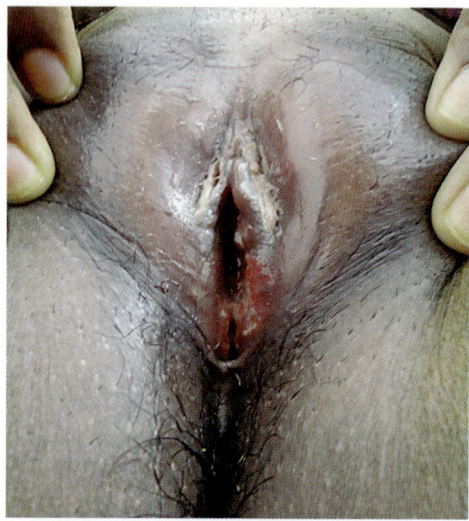

Figure 22: Herpes simplex presenting as painful genital ulcer

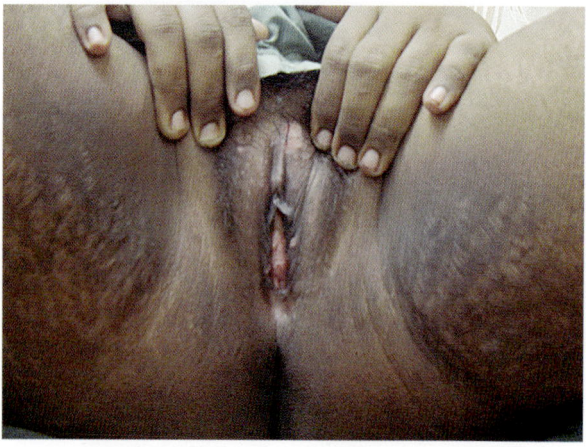

Figure 23: Infection by herpes simplex virus-1 and 2 in the same woman

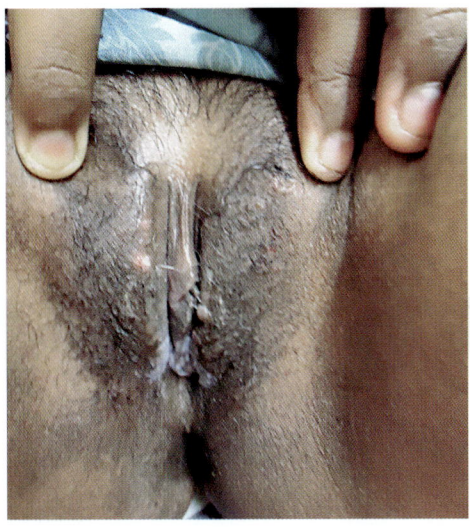

Figure 24: Genital herpes in a woman with vaginal discharge

Recurrences

After primary infection, the virus may be latent for months to years until a recurrence is triggered. Reactivation of HSV-2 in the lumbosacral ganglia leads to recurrences below the waist. Recurrent clinical outbreaks are milder and often preceded by a prodrome of pain, itching, tingling, burning, or paresthesia.

Asymptomatic viral shedding from genital skin may occur without symptoms or with unrecognized minor symptoms. The frequency of asymptomatic shedding is more common in those with type 2 genital herpes and in those who have been infected recently. Shedding is most likely to occur in the week before or after a recurrence.

Factors that increase the risk of transmission from mother to baby include the type of genital infection at the time of delivery (higher risk with active primary infection), active lesions, prolonged rupture of membranes, vaginal delivery, and an absence of transplacental antibodies. The mortality rate for neonates is extremely high (>80%), if untreated. Neonatal HSV usually manifests within the first 2 weeks

Genital Dermatoses

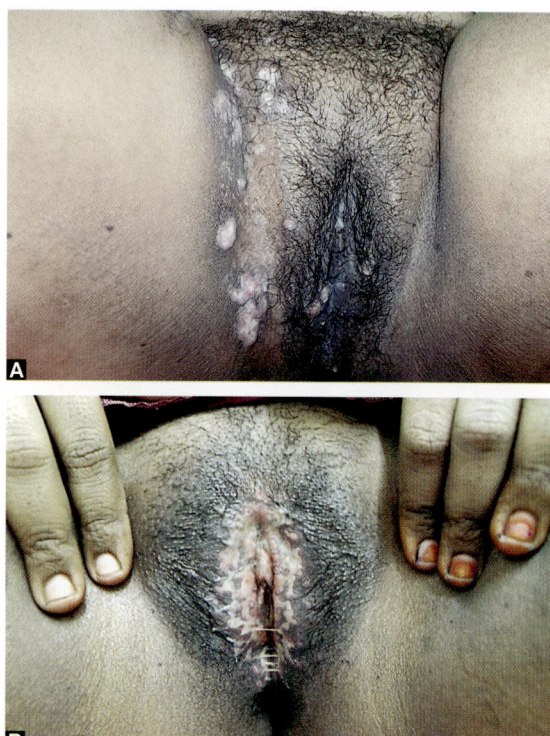

Figure 25: Herpes genitalis with secondary infection

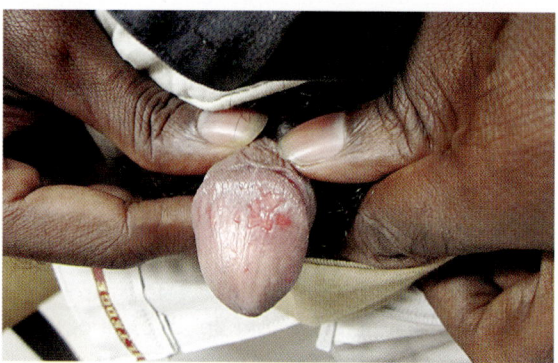

Figure 26: Herpes genitalis with multiple ulcers over glans penis

of life and clinically ranges from localized skin, mucosal, or eye infections to encephalitis, pneumonitis, and disseminated infection.

Sexual transmission of HIV is facilitated by genital ulcer disease due to disruption of the protective mucosal barrier and also the presence of increased numbers of activated CD4 T cells at the sites of infection. HIV infected persons have high rates of HSV-2 infection, ranging from 50 to 90% in different studies. They tend to have more severe, chronic, painful, and atypical lesions, as well as increased rates of asymptomatic genital shedding of HSV-2. Atypical presentations of herpes genitalis include deep progressive ulceration, hemorrhagic lesions, ecthyma like lesions, hyperkeratotic verrucous lesions resembling condylomata, and continuous and prolonged viral shedding.

Differential Diagnosis

The differential diagnosis includes primary syphilis, chancroid, Behcet's disease, aphthae, erythema multiforme, and candidiasis.

Investigations

Investigations should be routinely utilized to improve the diagnostic accuracy of genital herpes.

Tzanck smear can be helpful in the rapid diagnosis of genital herpes lesions (by identifying multinucleated giant cells), but it is less sensitive than viral culture. Immunofluorescence staining increases the sensitivity and specificity of a Tzanck smear preparation.

Histopathology is occasionally required in chronic herpes infection in HIV-infected individuals wherein morphology and clinical course are atypical.

Viral culture is the "gold standard" for HSV diagnosis. Cytopathic effects appear in 2–3 days after inoculation in human diploid fibroblast cultures or green monkey kidney cell cultures. Sensitivity of the tissue culture depends on the stage of clinical lesions; isolation is successful in about 80% of primary infections and in 25–50% of recurrent infections. Viral isolation is least successful in lesions that have begun to heal.

Herpes simplex virus direct detection tests include:
- Electron microscopy
- HSV antigen detection (immunoperoxidase tests, immunofluorescence, and enzyme immunoassay)
- Herpes simplex virus-deoxyribonucleic acid (HSV-DNA) detection (DNA hybridization)
- Herpes simplex virus-polymerase chain reaction (HSV-PCR).

Direct Fluorescent Antibody Test

Direct fluorescent antibody test (DFA) is used for the detection of HSV antigen in smear, tissues, or culture. The sensitivity of the DFA test for the detection of HSV in genital specimens varies between 70 and 90% of culture-positive specimens.

Rapid Assay

Herpes simplex virus antigen is extracted from the clinical specimen with a buffered solution. The extract is added to a test device and any antigen present is immobilized on a membrane. When treated peroxidase-labeled anti-HSV monoclonal antibody with substrate is added, a colored spot is obtained on the membrane. The sensitivity of this test is slightly lower than that of enzyme-linked immunosorbent assay (ELISA).

Herpes Simplex Virus-polymerase Chain Reaction

Polymerase chain reaction is more sensitive (four times) and faster than viral culture. Because the type of HSV infection affects prognosis and subsequent counseling, type-specific testing to distinguish HSV-1 from HSV-2 is recommended. Although PCR has been the diagnostic standard for HSV infections of the CNS, until now viral culture has been the test of choice for HSV genital infection. However, HSV-PCR, with its consistently and substantially higher rate of HSV detection, will likely replace viral culture as the gold standard for the diagnosis of genital herpes in people with active mucocutaneous lesions, regardless of anatomic location or viral type.

Serology

These tests detect antibodies to HSV in blood and it includes ELISA, complement fixation test, and Western blot. Accurate type-specific HSV serologic assays are based on the HSV-specific glycoprotein G2 (HSV-2) and glycoprotein G1 (HSV-1). Serology can rule out a prior HSV infection. HSV antibodies are absent in the acute stage but gradually appear, increase over subsequent weeks and persist for life. Seroconversion and a fourfold rise in antibody titers in acute and convalescent sera are seen after a true primary (first episode) infection. Seroconversion in pregnancy is associated with a high-risk of neonatal herpes. Recurrent episodes are rarely associated with an increase in antibody titers. Newer type-specific ELISAs can discriminate between HSV-1 and HSV-2 antibodies. Serology is useful in recurrent lesions, atypical lesions, healing lesions, culture-negative cases, unrecognized infection, and in evaluation of the sex partner. These tests may also be used to establish whether a herpetic outbreak is due to newly acquired infection for medicolegal purpose, and in HIV-infected individuals, for deciding on suppressive therapy. The most important application of serology is in the diagnosis of asymptomatic infections in transplant recipients and in patients receiving immunosuppressive drugs. Disadvantages of serological tests include false-negative results (due to delayed appearance of antibody or low sensitivity), false-positive results in low-risk populations, low purity of the recombinant glycoprotein G and the potential for cross-reactivity between glycoproteins G1 and G2 in ELISA, inability to determine the route of HSV acquisition (genital or oral), and difficulty in interpretation of results in HIV and other types of immunosuppressions. It must be remembered during interpretation of serological results that almost all HSV-2 infections are sexually acquired whereas HSV-1 antibodies indicate either an orolabial or a genital acquisition.

Treatment

Antiviral chemotherapy offers clinical benefits to the majority of symptomatic patients and is the mainstay of management.

Palliative measures like loose-fitting cotton underwears, cold compresses, saline bathing of the affected area, keeping the area dry and clean, and topical zinc cream application should be advised. Systemic antiviral drugs can partially control the signs and symptoms of herpes episodes when used to treat first clinical and recurrent episodes or when used as daily suppressive therapy. However, these drugs do not eradicate the latent virus. Currently, three drugs are approved for the treatment of genital herpes: acyclovir, valacyclovir, and famciclovir. Acyclovir is highly active against HSV-1, but slightly less active against HSV-2. The antiviral activity of acyclovir is due to the intracellular conversion of acyclovir, by viral thymidine kinase, to the monophosphate, with subsequent conversion by cellular kinases to diphosphate and the active triphosphate. This active form inhibits viral DNA synthesis and replication by inhibiting the herpes virus DNA polymerase enzyme as well as by being incorporated into the viral DNA causing premature DNA chain termination. The whole process is highly selective for infected cells because the initial activation needs viral thymidine kinase, and for the same reason, acyclovir has no activity against latent virus. Compared with acyclovir, penciclovir is 100–160 times less potent in inhibiting viral DNA polymerase but compensates for that by a longer half-life and higher intracellular concentration. Penciclovir inhibits viral DNA synthesis through irreversible and competitive inhibition of DNA polymerase rather than DNA chain termination. Penciclovir is not indicated for HSV-2 infections. Valacyclovir and famciclovir are prodrugs of acyclovir and penciclovir, respectively. They have enhanced absorption after oral administration and higher oral bioavailability, thereby allowing for lower dosage and lesser frequency of administration (oral bioavailability of acyclovir is 10–20% and that for valacyclovir is five times higher). Topical acyclovir preparations are less useful and are not recommended. Acyclovir resistance is most commonly due to mutation in the viral thymidine kinase and rarely due to mutation in viral DNA polymerase. In acyclovir resistance, valacyclovir and famciclovir are also ineffective. In spite of reports of treatment failure, resistance has never been a major problem in genital herpes.

Forcarnet inhibits viral DNA polymerase directly without requiring activation by viral thymidine kinase. Therefore, it is effective in acyclovir-resistant HSV infections. Foscarnet resistance is rare. Cidofovir, after activation by cellular kinases, inhibits viral DNA polymerase and is useful in acyclovir- and foscarnet-resistant cases. It is given intravenously (IV) once a week. Topical cidofovir 1% gel is also effective in acyclovir-resistant HSV infections.

First Episode Treatment

Many persons with first-episode herpes have severe or prolonged symptoms. Therefore, patients with initial genital herpes should receive antiviral therapy.

- Acyclovir 400 mg three times a day for 7-10 days
- Valacyclovir 1,000 mg twice a day for 7-10 days
- Famciclovir 250 mg three times a day for 7-10 days.

Episodic Therapy for Recurrent Genital Herpes

Effective episodic treatment of recurrent herpes requires initiation of therapy within 1 day of lesion onset or during the prodrome that precedes some outbreaks. The maximal viral replication occurs within 24 hours of the first prodromal symptom. Patient-initiated episodic therapy started during the onset of prodromal symptoms, which most patients can be easily taught to identify, is preferred by many clinicians because it takes advantage of the window period between onset of prodromal symptoms and clinically visible lesions of herpes (which is usually 12-24 hours). Episodic treatment with nucleoside analogs is usually given for 3-5 days. However, single-day patient-initiated episodic treatment (e.g., with famciclovir 1,000 mg twice daily or valacyclovir 2,000 mg twice daily) has been found to be a better option with better compliance and outcomes.

- Acyclovir 400 mg three times a day for 5 days
- Valacyclovir 500 mg twice a day for 3-5days
- Famciclovir 125 mg twice a day for 5 days.

Suppressive Therapy for Recurrent Genital Herpes

Suppressive therapy is indicated when recurrent genital herpes is frequent (≥6 recurrences in 1 year), severe, distressing or associated with distressing prodromes. Other indications are herpetic lesions in the last trimester, patients with psychological and psychosexual problems due to the infection, and immunocompromised patients. The risk of transmission of the virus to the sex partner is reduced as suppressive therapy reduces asymptomatic viral shedding.

Long-term antiviral prophylaxis may be started any time and continued for an unspecified duration. Safety and efficacy have been documented among patients receiving daily therapy with acyclovir for as long as 6 years and with valacyclovir or famciclovir for 1 year. Quality of life of patients with frequent recurrences is better in those who receive suppressive therapy than in those who receive episodic treatment. Long-term suppression is reported to reduce clinical outbreaks of genital herpes and subclinical shedding by 80 and 95%, respectively. The frequency of recurrent genital herpes outbreaks diminishes over time in many patients.

Breakthrough episodes during therapy should prompt one to look for poor compliance, need to adjust therapy, resistance or a mistaken diagnosis. A minimum of 3 months to 1 year of daily therapy is warranted for any efficacy. Some patients desire short-term suppression for a duration of 1 month. Annual evaluation is required and cessation of therapy (or drug holiday) should be discussed with patients who are well controlled for a long time. Some authors recommend that suppressive therapy should be discontinued after 12–24 months in order to assess the ongoing frequency of recurrences.

Valacyclovir appears to be somewhat better than famciclovir for the suppression of genital herpes and associated shedding. However, valacyclovir 500 mg once a day may be less effective than other acyclovir or valacyclovir regimens in patients with very frequent (>10 in a year) recurrences.

- Acyclovir 400 mg twice a day
- Valacyclovir 500 mg once a day for people with nine or fewer outbreaks per year
- Valacyclovir 500 mg twice a day or 1000 mg once a day for people with 10 or more outbreaks per year
- Famciclovir 250 mg twice a day.

Treatment of Severe Disease

Intravenous (IV) acyclovir therapy is recommended in patients who have severe HSV disease or complications that necessitate hospitalization (e.g., disseminated infection, pneumonitis or hepatitis) or CNS complications (e.g., meningitis or encephalitis). The recommended regimen is acyclovir 5–10 mg/kg body weight IV every 8 hours for 2–7 days or until clinical improvement is observed, followed by oral antiviral therapy to complete at least 10 days of total therapy.

Herpes Simplex Virus and Human Immunodeficiency Virus Coinfection

Antiretroviral therapy reduces the severity and frequency of symptomatic genital herpes, but frequent subclinical shedding still occurs. Suppressive or episodic therapy with oral antiviral agents is effective, in reducing HSV shedding, is safe and well tolerated, and may provide additional benefit by decreasing HIV-1 levels in the blood and genital tract. Treatment should be continued till all the lesions heal, which may take a significantly longer duration compared with genital herpes in the immunocompetent individuals. Some specialists suggest that HSV type-specific serology should be offered to HIV-positive persons during their initial evaluation and suppressive antiviral therapy should be considered in those who have HSV-2 infection. Acyclovir resistance is much higher (3.6–10.9%) in patients with HIV compared with immunocompetent hosts (<1%). The scenario did not change even after the introduction of highly active antiretroviral therapy (HAART). Cases of thrombotic microangiopathy reported earlier in the literature, occurring following valacyclovir therapy in the immunocompromised individuals, were related to a high dose of valacyclovir given for a prolonged duration. With the currently recommended dosage, such adverse effects are unlikely (patient on high-dose valacyclovir should, however, be monitored for such adverse effects). Valacyclovir has been FDA approved for use in HSV infections in HIV.

Genital Herpes in Pregnancy

The risk of neonatal transmission is low, if genital herpes occurs in the first and second trimester. However, patients with genital herpes after 34 weeks of gestation and those who have not completed at least 4 weeks of acyclovir therapy before delivery are at a high-risk of transmitting the infection to the neonates. Cesarean delivery is indicated for such cases, but it does not completely eliminate the risk. The best policy would be to continue acyclovir till delivery and perform cesarean section at full term. Elective cesarean delivery is especially indicated, if active HSV lesions are present during or within 2 weeks of labor.

Acyclovir, valacyclovir, and famciclovir are pregnancy category B drugs. Safety of these drugs in pregnancy has not been definitively established, but available data do not suggest major birth defects due to acyclovir. The benefits much outweigh the risk. Acylcovir attains good concentration in the fetus. Data regarding valacyclovir and famciclovir are limited. However, safety of acyclovir may be extended to valacylcovir as it is a prodrug of acyclovir.

Antiviral therapy (acyclovir 400 mg three times a day for 7–14 days or valacyclovir 1 g twice a day for 7–14 days) is recommended for women with symptomatic primary or first-episode HSV infection during pregnancy. Symptomatic recurrent HSV should be treated with acyclovir 400 mg three times a day for 5 days or valacyclovir 500 mg twice a day for 5 days. For women with frequent or severe recurrences, especially after the first trimester, daily suppressive therapy (acyclovir 400 mg three times a day or valacyclovir 500 mg twice a day) from 36 weeks of gestation till delivery may be indicated. Andrews et al. reported that administration of valacyclovir (500 mg twice a day) beginning at 36 weeks gestation till delivery in women with a history of recurrent genital HSV reduced the number of subsequent clinical HSV recurrences.

Prevention of neonatal herpes involves one or more of the following measures: serology for identifying those women at risk of acquiring new infection, recommendation of abstinence or protective condoms or antiviral prophylaxis in the context of a HSV-2-seropositive man and HSV-2-seronegative woman (seroincompatible), prophylactic antivirals from the 36th week of gestation in pregnant females at a high risk of HSV outbreaks during labor, antiviral treatment of HSV infections during late pregnancy, abstinence from oral sex in HSV-1-seroincompatible couples, thorough evaluation (including speculoscopy) for herpetic lesions during labor, avoiding exposure of the infant to herpetic lesions during delivery by performing cesarean section, providing occlusive dressing for nongenital lesions during labor, avoidance of iatrogenic trauma to the fetus, and refraining health care workers with visible herpetic lesions from providing postnatal care.

Neonatal Herpes

Infants suspected to have been exposed to HSV during birth should be followed carefully in consultation with a specialist and cultures of mucosal surfaces would be desirable. Some specialists recommend the use of acyclovir for infants born to women who acquired HSV near term.

Neonates delivered through an infected birth canal should be screened between 24 hours and 48 hours of age with viral cultures of the eyes, nasopharynx, mouth, and rectum. Treatment with systemic acyclovir should be started promptly. The recommended regimen for infants treated for known or suspected neonatal herpes is acyclovir 20 mg/kg body weight IV every 8 hours for 21 days for disseminated and CNS disease or for 14 days for disease limited to the skin and mucus membranes.

Drug Resistance

If lesions persist or recur in a patient receiving antiviral treatment, HSV resistance should be suspected and a viral isolate should be obtained for sensitivity testing. All acyclovir-resistant strains are resistant to valacyclovir, and the majorities are resistant to famciclovir. In the case of clinical resistance, virological studies with resistance testing should be carried out. This will help a clinician decide whether to give a high-dose oral or IV acyclovir, if the strain shows complete or intermediate sensitivity, or to switch to an alternative agent like foscarnet. Foscarnet, 40 mg/kg body weight IV every 8

Genital Dermatoses

hour until clinical resolution is attained, is frequently effective for the treatment of acyclovir-resistant genital herpes. Topical cidofovir gel 1% applied to the lesions once daily for five consecutive days might also be effective. A combination of multidrug therapy has also been tried in resistant HSV disease.

Counseling

Counseling of infected persons and their sex partners is critical to the management of genital herpes. The goal of counseling is to help patients cope with the infection and prevent sexual and perinatal transmission.

The following recommendations apply to counseling of persons with HSV infection:
- Explain and educate about the nature of genital herpes, the potential for recurrent episodes, asymptomatic viral shedding, and the risks of sexual transmission
- Explain the role of suppressive or episodic therapy in persons experiencing a first episode of genital herpes
- Encourage to inform the sex partners
- Explain the need to abstain from sexual activity with uninfected partners when lesions or prodromal symptoms are present
- Explain that latex condoms reduce the risk for genital herpes transmission
- Evaluate the sex partners, even in the absence of symptoms, by serology to identify serocompatibility
- Educate regarding neonatal herpes
- Seropositive but clinically asymptomatic patients should receive the same counseling message.

In addition, patients should be taught about the clinical manifestations and prodromal symptoms of genital herpes.

Prevention

- Prevention of genital herpes include the following measures: Sexual abstinence is the only method for absolute prevention of genital herpes

Sexually Transmitted Infection Affecting the Genitalia

- Contact should be avoided when active lesions are present. Avoid contact until re-epithelialization has occurred
- Use of condoms and spermicidal foams is recommended in patients who have a history of recurrent herpes genitalis
- Condoms are effective only if they cover all the lesions and are more effective at protecting susceptible females from HSV transmission than susceptible males
- If both partners had genital herpes, protective measures are not necessary, if both carry the same virus type and active lesions are not present
- Having herpes in one area is not protective against acquiring the infection in another location.

Vaccines

Vaccination, at least in theory, is the best method for preventing virus spread, but this strategy has been only marginally successful in genital herpes. The HSV candidate vaccines tested till now were mostly purified subunit vaccines and/or recombinant envelope glycoproteins [such as glycoprotein B (gB) and glycoprotein D (gD)]. In many experiments performed in mice, guinea pigs, and rabbits, clear-cut protection against acute virus challenge was demonstrated along with the reduction of the extent of latency. The immunotherapeutic effect of herpes vaccines seems less convincing. However, the introduction of new adjuvants, which shift the cytokine production of helper T-cells toward the stimulation of cytotoxic T-cells, reveals a promising development.

Recently, the results of two controlled trials of an HSV type 2 (HSV-2) gD vaccines revealed that vaccination reduced the rate of acquisition of genital herpes disease, but it did so only among HSV-seronegative women. The vaccine did not reduce the risk of disease among men and did not add to the protection provided by a previous HSV-1 infection in women.

Future Trends

Helicase-primase inhibitors are new non-nucleoside antivirals that target the helicase-primase complex critically involved in HSV DNA replication. Results from animal studies are encouraging. They may prove to be the new generation of anti-HSV drugs with improved efficacy, less toxicity, better cost-effectiveness, and more convenient administration. A study using BAY 57-1293, a helicase-primase inhibitor, in animal models of ocular HSV-1 infection showed that it is more effective than valacyclovir with a good safety profile.

Zhang et al. tested a novel needle-free mucosal vaccine containing synthetic peptide epitopes of HSV-2 extended with an agonist of toll-like receptor 2 (TLR-2) that are abundantly expressed by dendritic and epithelial cells of the vaginal mucosa. After intravaginal inoculation, there was the development of protective immunity (local and systemic CD8+ T cells response) against HSV-2. A new microbicide product named VivaGel (containing SPL7013 as the active ingredient) has been showing promising efficacy and safety in initial animal and human studies.

METHODS OF SPECIMEN COLLECTION FOR THE DIAGNOSIS OF SEXUALLY TRANSMITTED INFECTIONS

Many of the landmark discoveries with regard to the etiology, pathogenesis, and epidemiology of STIs occurred with the use of various diagnostic techniques many years ago. However, the concept of providing comprehensive laboratory services for the diagnosis of STIs has surfaced relatively recently. The correct method of specimen collection helps in achieving desirable goals in the laboratory diagnosis of STIs. If simple precautions are taken, it will avoid spurious results. The collection of specimens and use of the appropriate swab and transport media are vital in the success of tissue culture.

Principles to be followed while collecting specimens:
- Communication with laboratory staff to discuss collection, transport, and testing of specimens
- All procedures should be performed while wearing appropriate protective gear

- Avoid contamination by indigenous commensal flora
- Adequate volumes of each specimen should be collected
- All specimens should be labeled correctly with the patient's name, hospital number and source, date and time of collection
- Leakproof containers should be used
- Optimal transport conditions should be followed as many of the organisms are fastidious.

The common laboratory diagnostic procedures that can be done in the outpatient department are:
- Dark-field microscopy for syphilis
- Gram staining for gonorrhea, nongonococcal urethritis, chancroid, and bacterial vaginosis
- Tzanck smear for herpes genitalis, donovanosis, and MC
- Wet mount for trichomoniasis
- KOH wet mount for candidiasis
- Bubo aspiration and smear for LGV and chancroid.

Dark-Field Microscopy

Dark-field examination is most productive in primary, secondary, and early congenital syphilis, when moist lesions containing large numbers of treponemes (e.g., chancres, condylomata lata, umbilical cord or mucous patches) are present. Aspirate from enlarged regional lymph nodes and cervical and vaginal specimens can also be used, but oral lesions are avoided as even an experienced observer may find it difficult to differentiate *T. pallidum* from saprophytic spirochetes. The specimen for dark-field microscopy consists of serous fluid that contains *T. pallidum*, but should be free of erythrocytes, other organisms, and tissue debris.

Method of Specimen Collection for Dark-field Microscopy

Observe universal safety precautions.
- To clean the lesion, only if it is encrusted or obviously contaminated
- Use only tap water or physiological saline (without antibacterial additives). Antiseptics or soaps should not be used as they may

Genital Dermatoses

kill the treponemes. Use minimal amounts of liquid for cleaning as large amounts may dilute and reduce the yield of the organisms
- Gently abrade the lesion with dry gauze, wipe away any blood-stained exudate, and apply gentle pressure until only clear serum exudes
- Collect the specimen directly on a cover slip or a clean glass slide by pressing directly onto the lesion
- For cervical and vaginal lesions, identify the lesion by speculum examination, clean with saline; abrade with a gauze pad held in suitable forceps. Collect the serous exudates using a bacteriological loop or Pasteur pipette and transfer to a slide
- If material is not sufficient, mix with a drop of saline
- Seal the edges of the cover slip with petroleum jelly
- Examine immediately
- If negative at first, dark-field examination should be repeated daily for at least three consecutive days.

Gram Staining

Sterile cotton, calcium alginate, Dacron rayon or polyethylene terephthalate (PET) swabs with plastic or aluminum shaft or bacteriological loop can be used for collecting the specimen. Gram staining is useful for the diagnosis of gonococcal and nongonococcal urethritis, mucopurulent cervicitis, chancroid, bacterial vaginosis, and candidal infections.

Gonorrhea

The choice of the specimen depends on the age, sex, sexual habits, and clinical presentation of the patient.
- Heterosexual men: Urethra, and first void urine (FVU)
- Homosexual men: Urethra, rectum, and oropharynx
- Women
    - Primary site: Endocervical canal
    - Secondary sites: Urethra, vagina, rectum, and oropharynx

Two swabs should always be collected, one for direct microscopy and one for culture. Transport media should be used, if the laboratory is not in the vicinity of the clinic.

Method of Collection of the Specimen

In men the method of collection of specimen is as follows:
- Urethral swab:
  - Collect specimen at least 2 hours after urination as voiding decreases the amount of exudates
  - Retract the prepuce, clean the tip of the meatus with normal saline and collect the pus directly onto a glass slide or sterile swab in case of frank urethral discharge
  - If no urethral discharge is seen, milk or strip the urethra from the root of the penis to the glans and collect the discharge as above
  - If no discharge is obtained, insert a sterile cotton tipped or thin calcium alginate swab with a flexible wire shaft or a bacteriological loop 2-3 cm into the urethra and rotate for 5-10 seconds
  - If there is no evidence of urethritis on examination, but there is a history of contact, ask the patient to hold the urine overnight and then milk or strip the urethra and collect the discharge, if any. If no discharge is obtained, insert a swab and collect the specimen as above.
- Urine:
  - The first 10-15 mL of the early morning first void urine is collected in a sterile plastic container with a wide mouth and processed immediately.

In women the method of specimen collection is as follows:
- Endocervical swab:
  - Cervical specimens are not collected in prepubertal girls since GC in this age group involves the vagina and not the cervix
  - No antiseptics, analgesics or lubricants should be applied
  - A sterile vaginal speculum moistened with warm water is inserted in the vagina and the ectocervix is visualized
  - After cleaning the ectocervix using forceps with a sterile cotton swab, insert a sterile swab 2-3 cm into the endocervical canal, rotate and move from side to side for 5-10 seconds and withdraw.

Genital Dermatoses

- Urethral swab:
  - Same method as for men, except that the urethra is massaged against the pubic symphysis from its proximal end towards the meatus, if no pus is visible.
- Vaginal swab:
  - Prepubertal or unmarried girls and women who have undergone hysterectomy
  - Vaginal swab or vaginal tampon may be used to obtain the specimen
  - Using a speculum, swab the posterior fornix with a sterile swab in women
  - Collect the specimen without a speculum in prepubertal girls.

In both sexes the method of specimen collection is as follows:
- Rectal swab:
  - If recent anal intercourse is admitted, a proctoscope is inserted, followed by a swab stick inserted 3 cm into the anal canal, rotating it for 10 seconds to collect the exudates or mucus or muco-pus from the crypts just inside the anal ring. If fecal contamination occurs, discard and collect a fresh specimen.
- Pharyngeal swab:
  - If orogenital contact with an infected person is suspected, a specimen is collected from the tonsillar crypts and the bed of the pharynx in both sexes.

Nongonococcal Urethritis or Cervicitis

- Specimen is collected in the same manner as for gonorrhea, but as discharge may be scanty, samples are collected after holding the urine for 3-4 hours.

Chancroid

- Specimens are collected from the undermined edge or the base of the ulcer. Organisms are usually demonstrable in the aspirate from an intact bubo
- Wipe the lesion with saline gauze followed by dry gauze (thorough cleaning not essential) to remove the superficial debris and crusts. Roll a sterile swab in one direction beneath the undermined edge

Sexually Transmitted Infection Affecting the Genitalia

of the ulcer. Re-roll the swab in the reverse direction at 180° on a clean glass slide to maintain the arrangement of the bacteria
- Use appropriate transport media for cultures.

Bacterial Vaginosis
- Specimen is collected from the posterior or lateral wall of the vagina with a sterile swab soaked in saline.

Tzanck Smear or Giemsa Stain
Giemsa stain can be used in the diagnosis of genital herpes, MC, donovanosis, and chancroid.

Genital Herpes
- Scrapings from blister or vesicle or ulcer base for Tzanck smear
- Vesicle (<72-hours-old): Open with an 18 g hypodermic needle on one side, drain the fluid, fold the roof back, and scrape the undersurface of the roof and floor with a curette or scalpel. The vesicle fluid may be sent for culture, where facilities are available
- Ulcer: Cotton-tipped swab on a wire shaft is used
- Women with genital herpes: Swab ectocervix and junction of ecto and endo cervix for Tzanck smear and culture
- Asymptomatic women: Use a single swab premoistened with saline to rub the clitoral hood, labia minora and majora, perineum, and perianal region for culture
- Men without vesicles: Swab urethra and meatus for Tzanck smear and culture
- Asymptomatic neonates: Use swabs premoistened with saline; one each from the conjunctiva, mouth, around the lips, external auditory canal, umbilicus, axillae, and groins for culture.

Donovanosis
- Wipe the lesion with saline gauze, followed by dry gauze. Remove a small piece of tissue from the border of a well-defined ulcer using a curette or forceps or edge of a safety razor blade. Place this specimen on a clean grease-free microscopic glass slide and crush the specimen between two clean slides (Rajam and Rangiah method)

Genital Dermatoses

- Alternatively, a crush biopsy specimen may be used (Greenblatt and Barfield method)
- Impression smears from the lower surface of the biopsy specimen may also be used
- The specimen is air-dried and stained with Giemsa or Leishman stain.

Molluscum Contagiosum

- Compress the lesion to extrude the cheesy material or use a small curette to remove the top of a papule
- Crush the specimen between two clean grease-free microscopic slides and stain.

KOH Mount

This test may be used for the diagnosis of genital candidiasis and bacterial vaginosis.

- Under speculum examination, the specimen is collected with a cotton or polyester swab from the wall of the posterior fornix. The skin surrounding the genitals is also scrapped
- In men, the swab is moistened with saline and the glans surface is scrapped
- The specimen is mixed with a drop of 10–20% KOH on a glass slide, covered with a cover slip and examined under high power (40 x lens).

Wet Mount

This is a simple diagnostic procedure commonly used to visualize trichomonads, but can also demonstrate candida and organisms responsible for bacterial vaginosis.

- Under speculum examination, the vaginal swab is collected from the posterior fornix using a sterile swab or bacteriological loop. In men, the urethra is sampled with a cotton wool or polyester swab
- The specimen is mixed with 1 mL of body-temperature saline in a test tube or directly mixed with a drop of normal saline on a slide.

Using warmed saline or warming the slide enhances the motility of the trichomonads.

Bubo Aspiration

Nonfluctuant Bubo (for Syphilis)

In cases in which an antibiotic or other antiseptic lotion or cream has been applied on the primary sore or in which the sore is healing or is hidden in the terminal portion of the urethra or under a phimotic prepuce, diagnostic puncture of lymph nodes is particularly useful. By this technique, 0.1 mL of sterile normal saline is injected into an enlarged regional lymph node before aspiration. The enlarged node is first steadied between finger and thumb with the skin stretched over it. A hypodermic needle attached to a small syringe containing 0.1 mL saline is introduced through the skin along the long axis of the node and plunged well into its body. Movement of the syringe and needle in various directions will confirm that the needle is in the correct position. The saline is then injected into the node and after further movement of the needle to encourage flow of lymph, aspiration is performed. The fluid material so obtained is used for dark-field microscopy.

Fluctuant Bubo (for Lymphogranuloma venereum and Chancroid)

- The patient is made to lie in the supine position and the area is painted with (povidone iodine)
- The bubo is aspirated from the non-dependent fluctuant part with a 16–18 g needle with a 10 or 20 mL syringe till most of the fluid is aspirated.

Method of Specimen Collection for Immunofluorescence

Immunofluorescence techniques are used primarily in the diagnosis of syphilis and herpes genitalis. For the detection of *T. pallidum* (direct fluorescent antibody test-*T. pallidum* "DFA-Tp"), lesion exudates, tissues, body fluids or secretions are taken onto slides, dried and fixed with acetone, and then stained. For herpes genitalis, the specimen is directly taken from the lesions or centrifuged deposits from transport media containing the specimen. For chancroid, gonorrhea, chlamydia, and trichomoniasis, immunofluorescence has been described but is not routinely used.

Methods for Polymerase Chain Reaction

The type of specimen taken is less critical for PCR and neither refrigeration nor rapid transport is required. PCR and LCR give good results even in first-catch urine samples or self-administered vaginal swabs for *Chlamydia trachomatis*. The combined detection of gonorrhea and *Chlamydia trachomatis* has been achieved on urethral discharge. Multiplex genital ulcer PCR can detect *T. pallidum, Haemophilus ducreyi,* and HSV types 1 and 2 from genital sore exudate or tissue.

Transport Media for Culture

In general, transport must be as rapid as possible, avoiding excesses of temperature. The ideal transportation temperature for Chlamydia (sucrose phosphate transport media in cryo vials) is 4°C, whereas ambient room temperature is recommended for *N. gonorrhoeae* [nutritive media containing carbon dioxide-Transgrow or John E. Martin biological environmental chamber (JEMBEC) or non-nutritive media-Stuarts or Amies]. Plastic or metal shafts are better than cotton-tipped swabs on wooden sticks for obtaining the specimen for chlamydia and mycoplasma. For herpes, the specimen is to be placed in 1 ml of viral transport medium and stored at 4°C till inoculation into tissue culture media. For storage more than 48 hours, the sample may be frozen at 70°C. Whittington or Kupferberg medium is used as transport medium for *Trichomonas vaginalis*.

CHAPTER 7

Genital Infections Other Than Sexually Transmitted Diseases

Infectious non-venereal diseases of the anogenital region are caused by viruses, fungi, bacteria, and *Mycobacteria*. Some infections are part of the generalized infection, while some are limited to the mucosa and skin genital area. Varicella and hand-foot- and -mouth disease are common diseases of childhood that can involve the genital skin. Candidiasis, dermatophytosis, erythrasma, folliculitis, erysipelas, and malakoplakia can be localized to the genital area, and it is of interest to note that these are more common in diabetics. Perianal abscess and lupus vulgaris affecting the perianal area, can sometimes pose diagnostic challenge.

TINEA CRURIS

Tinea cruris is a pruritic, superficial, fungal infection of the groin and adjacent skin. It is also known as "dhobi's itch" or "jock itch."

Etiology and Pathogenesis

The most common etiologic agents for tinea cruris include *Trichophyton rubrum* and *Epidermophyton floccosum*; less commonly *T. mentagrophytes* and *T. verrucosum* are involved. Tinea cruris is a contagious infection transmitted by fomites, such as contaminated towels or by autoinoculation from a reservoir on the hands or feet (tinea manuum, tinea pedis, and tinea unguium).

Genital Dermatoses

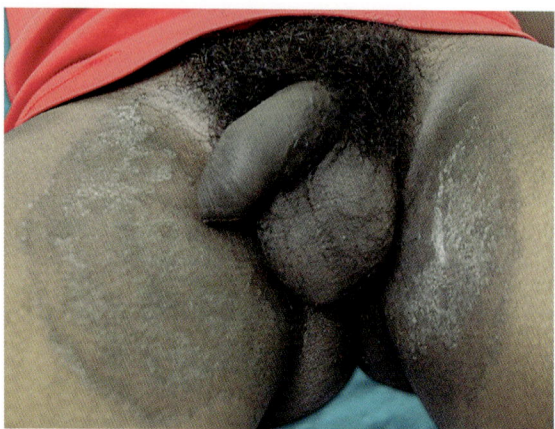

Figure 1: Dermatophytosis showing pigmented scaly plaque with raised border over groin, thighs

The etiologic agents in tinea cruris produce keratinases, which allow invasion of the cornified cell layer of the epidermis. The host immune response may prevent deeper invasion. Risk factors for initial tinea cruris infection or re-infection include wearing tight-fitting undergarments. It is three times more common in men than in women.

Clinical Features

Patients present with diffuse bilateral erythema and scaling along the inguinal folds. A raised border typical of tinea infection is usually present (Fig. 1). The eruption may extend along the perineum up the gluteal cleft. Involvement of the scrotum is distinctly uncommon and another diagnosis should be considered with extensive scrotal involvement.

Diagnosis

Microscopic examination of a potassium hydroxide (KOH) wet mount of scales is diagnostic in tinea cruris.

Wood lamp examination may be helpful to exclude erythrasma, which reveals coral red fluorescence of the affected area.

Differential Diagnosis

Candidiasis is more common in females and lesions do not have a distinct raised margin. Pityriasis versicolor and erythrasma may be localized to the groins, but are asymptomatic and there is no central clearance. Intertrigo and flexural psoriasis are other differential diagnosis.

Treatment

Clinical cure of an uncomplicated tinea cruris infection usually can be achieved using topical antifungal agents of the imidazole or allylamine family. Consider patients, unable to use topical treatments consistently or with extensive or recalcitrant infection, as candidates for systemic administration of antifungal therapy.

ERYTHRASMA

Erythrasma is a chronic, scaly dermatosis affecting the body flexures and intertriginous areas of adults, caused by a diphtheroid termed as *Corynebacterium minutissimum*. The bacterium is a lipophilic, gram-positive, nonspore-forming, aerobic, and catalase-positive diphtheroid. *C minutissimum* ferments glucose, dextrose, sucrose, maltose, and mannitol.

The typical appearance of erythrasma is well-demarcated, brown-red macular patches. The skin has a wrinkled appearance with fine scales (Fig. 2). Infection, commonly, is located over inner thighs, crural region, scrotum, and toe webs. Folds of skin in obese persons and flexures like axilla and inframammary region in females are other common sites of involvement (Fig. 3). Heat, humidity, hydration, poor hygiene, obesity, and diabetes mellitus predispose an individual to this disease. In obese and diabetics, erythrasma and candidal intertrigo can co-exist (Fig. 4).

Corynebacterium minutissimum shows coral red fluorescence under Wood's light due to water soluble coproporphyrin III produced by the organisms. Hence, washing the area will remove the fluorescence.

Genital Dermatoses

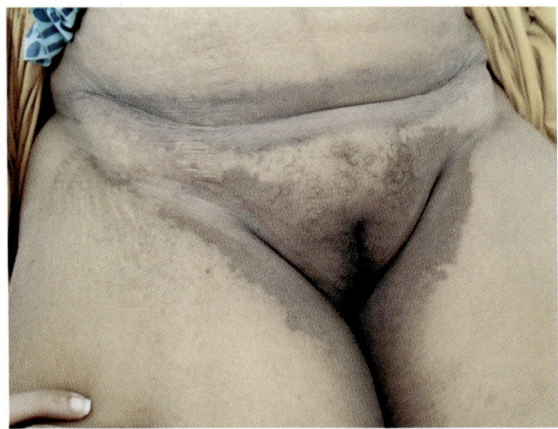

Figure 2: Well demarcated, brown-red patches of erythrasma over pubic region, lower abdomen & groin

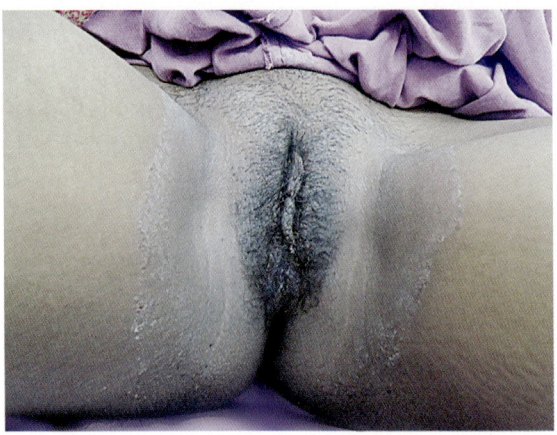

Figure 3: Dermatophytosis of the genital skin and groins, Note the advancing margin

Treatment

Topical fusidic acid or imidazoles can be effective, but systemic erythromycin or tetracycline should be the drug of choice, especially in an extensive case as they also reduce the incidence of relapses.

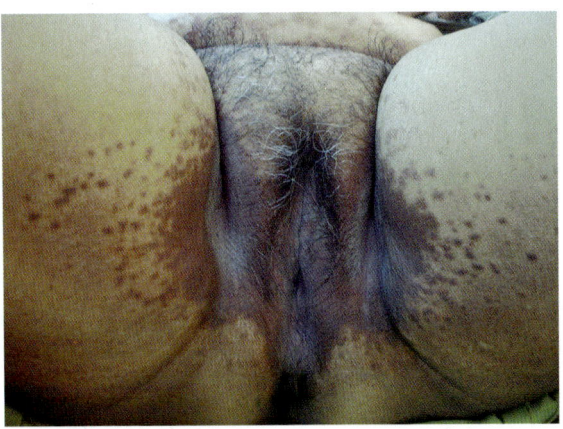

Figure 4: Erythrasma with candidal intertrigo in a diabetic

CANDIDAL BALANITIS

Balanitis refers to the inflammation of the glans, while posthitis refers to the inflammation of the foreskin. Inflammation of both of these is known as balanoposthitis. The skin of the glans penis, especially in the uncircumcised, may sometimes be colonized by candida asymptomatically. Candida species account for 30–35% cases of infectious balanitis. Candidiasis of the glans penis is more common in diabetic uncircumcised patients and in those whose sexual partner has candidal vulvovaginitis. However, oral and anal transmission is equally important. Mild cases present with small popular lesions over the glans a few hours after intercourse. Not all cases of candidal balanitis are sexually transmitted. Even children can develop candidal balanitis (Fig. 5). As the condition progresses, pustules and vesicles are formed that rupture to form an irregular, fringed edge. A little soreness or irritation is noted. Some cases may resolve spontaneously, while in others the condition continues to be intermittent. Chronic and severe cases show similar inflammatory changes that become persistent over the glans and prepuce, and cause considerable soreness. Candidal intertrigo of the groins may co-exist.

Genital Dermatoses

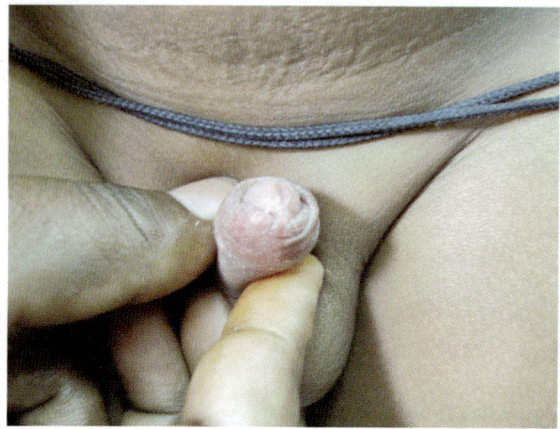

Figure 5: Candidal balanitis showing erythema and fissuring

Treatment

Recommended Regimens

- Clotrimazole topical cream applied twice a day for 10–14 days
- Miconazole topical cream applied twice a day for 10–14 days
- Econazole 1% twice daily.

Alternative Regimens

- Topical imidazole with 1% hydrocortisone
- Fluconazole 150 mg stat orally in recalcitrant cases or with diabetes.

VULVOVAGINAL CANDIDIASIS AND VULVOVAGINITIS

Vulvovaginal candidiasis (VVC) is part of a group of infections termed the superficial fungal infections. These can be classified as complicated or uncomplicated, sporadic or recurrent. Some patients are difficult to diagnose, and may not respond to standard therapies. These patients suffer from recurrent or chronic VVC. Recurrent VVC is defined as more than four episodes of VVC within a 12-month period. Patients normally present with a white, cheesy discharge and vulvovaginal itching. Clinically, it presents as erythema and edema of the vestibule and of the labia majora and minora. The erythema may extend to the thighs and perineum. Thrush patches are usually found loosely adherent to the vulva. A thick, white, curd-like vaginal discharge is usually present. Candidal vaginitis is more itchy, while bacterial vaginits is more painful. When there is super added herpes infection, patient may complain of pain (Figs 6 to 9). During normal pregnancy, candidiasis is frequently encountered without significant risk for the fetus. Nevertheless, VVC may occasionally jeopardize an otherwise successful pregnancy. VVC could represent a risk factor for candidemia in preterm neonate during the normal partum. Early detection, early diagnosis, and appropriate treatment may improve the women, pregnant or nonpregnant and neonate clinical conditions. Recommendations for vulvovaginitis diagnosis included speculum examination and microscopic examination of slide from vaginal exudates to look for protozoal (*Trichomonas vaginalis*), bacterial (*Gardnerella vaginalis*), or fungal (*Candida* spp.) agents, followed by vaginal fluid specimen culture to confirm the diagnosis.

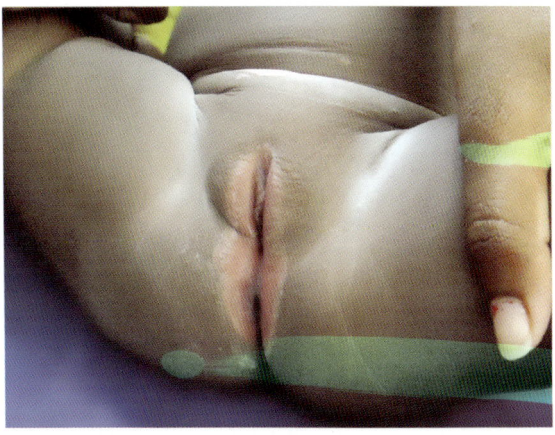

Figure 6: Candidal vaginitis in a child

Genital Dermatoses

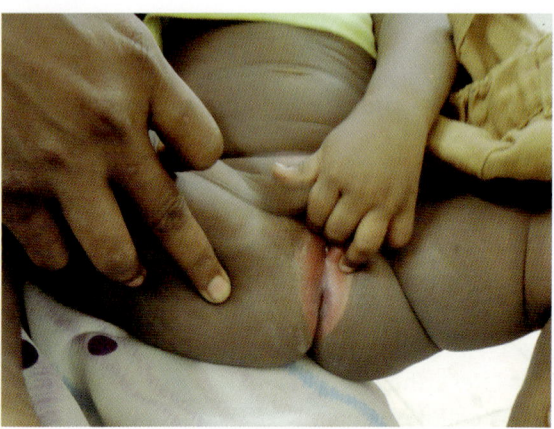

Figure 7: Candidal vaginitis is more itchy while bacterial vaginitis is more painful

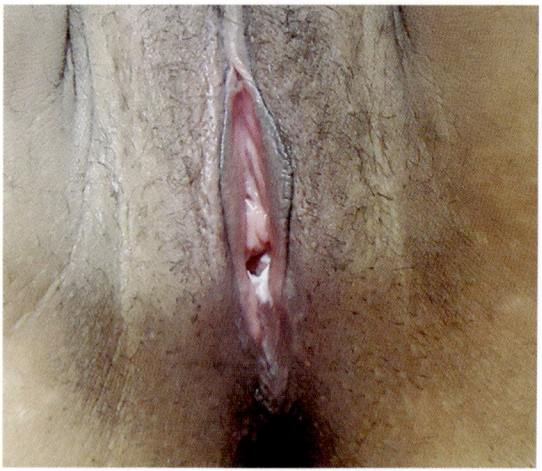

Figure 8: Candidal vaginitis in a pregnant woman

Treatment

Intravaginal and oral therapy provides equally effective treatment for vaginal candidiasis. Treatment with azoles results in relief of

Genital Infections Other Than Sexually Transmitted Diseases

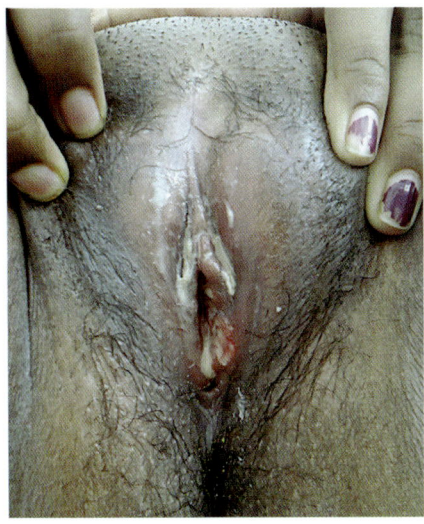

Figure 9: Candidal vaginitis with Herpes simplex

symptoms and negative cultures among 80-90% of patients after treatment is completed, whether administered orally or topically. Only topical preparations should be used during pregnancy. Overall standard single-dose treatments are as effective as longer courses. In a severely symptomatic attack, there is proven to be better symptomatic benefit in repeating fluconazole 150 mg after 3 days. This does not affect relapse rates.

Oral preparations include:
- Fluconazole 150 mg as a single dose
- Itraconazole 200 mg twice daily for 1 day.

Intravaginal treatments include:
- Clotrimazole vaginal tablet 500 mg or 200 mg once daily for 3 days
- Miconazole vaginal ovule 1200 mg as a single dose or 400 mg once daily for 3 days
- Econazole vaginal pessary 150 mg as a single dose.

There are a number of other intravaginal preparations available. These are now all either azoles or of limited availability, e.g., nystatin or unlicensed. Topical treatment to the vulva is of no proven added benefit to intravaginal treatment, but some patients prefer this.

Genital Dermatoses

Where itch is a significant symptom, a hydrocortisone containing topical preparation may provide more rapid symptomatic relief.

For practical purpose, the terms vulvitis, vaginitis, and vulvovaginitis often are used interchangeably for inflammatory conditions of the lower female genital tract. Vulvitis may occur alone or accompanied by a secondary vaginitis. Conversely, primary vaginal infection in a child, may cause secondary vulvitis due to maceration caused by vaginal discharge. Vulvovaginitis presents as genital irritation, pain, and dysuria with or without vaginal discharge. (Fig. 10).

Vaginitis in the newborn is most frequently caused by maternal vaginal micro-organisms acquired during labor. Pediatric inflammatory vulvovaginitis is mainly caused by pathogens of the upper respiratory tract and the most common risk factor for this infection is to have suffered an upper respiratory tract infection in the previous month, while vaginitis in children is frequently caused by group A and group B *Streptococcus*, less frequently by *Escherichia coli, Haemophilus influenzae,* and rarely by *Enterobius vermicularis*. Vulvovaginitis is the most common gynecological problem in prepubertal girls.

Bacterial vaginitis in postmenopausal women is most frequently caused by overgrowth of bacteria from the nearby gastrointestinal

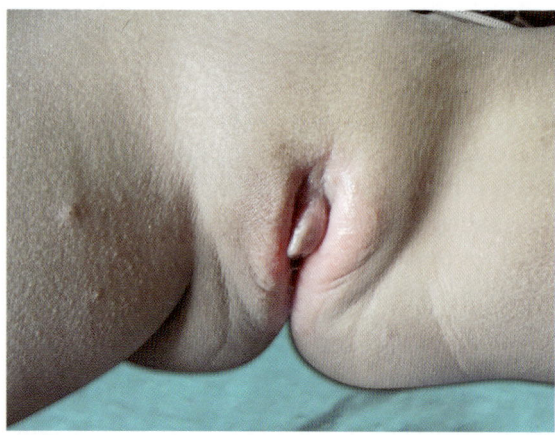

Figure 10: Bacterial vaginitis in an infant

tract and/or bacterial vaginosis (BV)-associated organisms. Evaluation of these infections commonly involves aerobic culture and specific treatment along with systemic or topical estrogen treatment in women lacking estrogen.

TRICHOMYCOSIS PUBIS

The name is a misnomer, since it is not a fungal infection. The causative organism associated with most cases is *Corynebacterium tenuis*, which prefers the moist microenvironment of the inguinal regions. It is characterized by the appearance of asymptomatic, yellow, red and black, dirty-looking, small concretions usually on the hair shaft. Sweat in the region tends to be colored, similarly. Lesions present in the inguinal region, often on the scrotum but occasionally on the base of the shaft of the penis. Lesions can be associated with erythema and itching, and superinfection with dermatophytes has been noted.

The concretions are colonies of coryneform bacteria. These bacteria colonize and invade the hair shaft surface and penetrate into the cuticle. The colonies adhere to the shaft by a cement substance, the nature of which is not well understood, but is probably a glucon analogue produced by coryneforms.

Treatment

Management involves clipping the axillary hair and applying 1% aqueous formalin. Antimicrobial creams such as benzoic acid are also helpful. Regular use of antiperspirants such as anhydrous aluminum chloride is recommended.

FOLLICULITIS

Folliculitis usually caused by *Staphylococcus aureus* is common in the follicle-rich genital region. Typically, patients have several 1–2 mm pustules, each centered around a hair follicle. Careful examination may show a hair follicle, extending out of the pustule. Note the lesions are not grouped nor are they usually unilateral like genital herpes. Deeper involvement can lead to furunculosis, when

Genital Dermatoses

the lesion is bigger and more painful (Fig. 11). Folliculitis can occur anywhere on the genitals, though less common on the distal penis due to absence of follicles. Heat and sweat are aggravating factors. Patients may give a history of a new exercise routine or wearing synthetic jogging pants that retain perspiration. Patients will respond to topical or oral antibiotics directed toward *S. aureus*. A mainstay of treatment is antibacterial soap.

MALAKOPLAKIA

Malakoplakia is an inflammatory condition presenting as a plaque or a nodule that usually affects the genitourinary tract, but may rarely involve the skin. Malakoplakia was first described in the early 1900s as yellow soft plaques that were seen on the mucosa of the urinary bladder. Cutaneous malakoplakia is rare, but presents in patients who are immunocompromised and have defects in macrophage function. Lesions are yellow-to-pink papules, but they can present as nodules or ulcerations and are often diagnosed only after biopsy.

Microscopically, malakoplakia is characterized by the presence of foamy histiocytes with distinctive basophilic inclusions, which are known as Michaelis-Gutmann bodies.

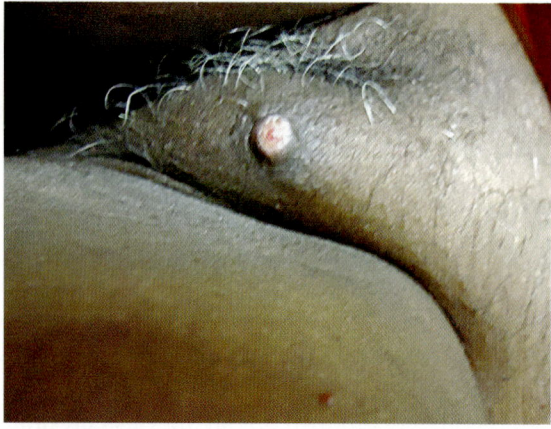

Figure 11: Folliculitis of the genital skin

ERYSIPELAS

Erysipelas is a bacterial skin infection involving the upper dermis that characteristically extends into the superficial cutaneous lymphatics (Fig. 12). It is a tender, intensely erythematous, and indurated plaque with a sharply-demarcated border. It's well-defined margins and presence of vesicles in the advancing margin can help differentiate it from cellulitis. Genital erysipelas is caused by group A hemolytic streptococci. The role of *Staphylococcus aureus*, and specifically methicillin-resistant *S. aureus* (MRSA), remains controversial. Lymphatic obstruction or edema and immunocompromised state like diabetes and HIV infection can predispose to the disease. Presence of genital erysipelas should arouse a suspicion to identify diseases, such as folliculitis and furunculosis of the genital skin.

Treatment

General measures like bed rest and adequate fluid intake should be advised. Apart from analgesics and antipyretics, penicillin is the standard therapy for typical erysipelas. Erythromycin, cephalexin, and dicloxacillin are other drugs useful in treating erysipelas.

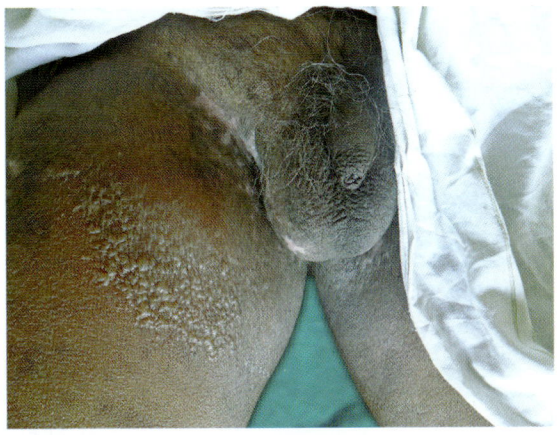

Figure 12: Erysipelas of the thigh extending to the groin and genitals

Genital Dermatoses

PERIANAL ABSCESS

A perianal abscess refers to collection of pus, outside the anus. Inciting factors include, infection of an anal fissure, sexually transmitted infections, and blocked perianal glands. When bacteria gains entry through a tear in the lining of the rectum or anus, it leads to formation of an abscess. This abscess increases in size, following the plane of least resistance and spread towards the surface, creating a perianal abscess. Occasionally, the infection can lead to ischiorectal or supralevator abscesses. Immunocompromised states, such as diabetes, and inflammatory bowel disease, such as Crohn's disease should be excluded (Fig. 13).

Painful swelling in the perianal area with or without pus discharge is the presenting complaint. However, discharge of pus is not necessary for diagnosis. The cardinal signs of inflammation, namely pain, fever, redness, swelling, and loss of function will be typically present. History should be taken and per rectal examination along with procto-sigmoidoscopy should be done to rule out conditions, such as Crohn's disease.

Treatment

Prompt incision and drainage of the abscess is usually the preferred treatment. When Crohn's disease is suspected, appropriate

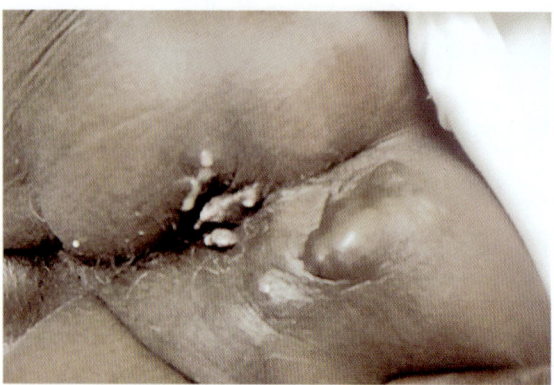

Figure 13: Perianal abscess with multiple sites of pus discharge, should consider Crohn's disease

treatment should be given. However, the role of surgical intervention in the treatment of patients with Crohn's disease is controversial. Complications of surgery include systemic infection, anal fistula formation, recurrence, and scarring.

TUBERCULOSIS

Tuberculosis (TB) of the genital tract is a common cause for infertility in females. However, cutaneous TB of the skin involving ano-genital area is not uncommon. TB verrucosa cutis, lupus vulgaris (LV), and scrofuloderma are the common cutaneous TB that are seen in the genital area.

Tuberculosis verrucosa cutis results from direct inoculation of TB bacilli into the skin in person who has been previously infected with *Mycobacteria*. It starts as rough papule or plaque, and enlarges to a purplish or brownish-red warty growth. Gluteal skin is commonly affected site in the ano-genital area. Lesions may persist for years, but can rarely clear up even without treatment.

Lupus vulgaris is the most common form of cutaneous TB resulting from hematogeneous or lymphatic spread of *Mycobacteria* from an endogeneous focus in a previously sensitized host with a high level of cell-mediated immunity. LV, classically presents as a solitary, asymptomatic plaque with an atrophic centre and an infiltrated, serpiginous, or polycyclic red-brown border (Fig. 14). The plaque is formed by coalescence of soft, friable, and gelatinous papules. These papules give the appearance of apple jelly on *in vitro* pressure(diascopy). Misdiagnosis and delayed treatment of LV sometimes occur because of the variations in the clinical presentation and the low rate of positive cultures. Annular form of LV can easily be misdiagnosed for dermatophyte infection and treatment delayed.

Scrofuloderma also called 'TB colliquativa cutis' affects children and young adults. Clinical features include discharging sinus overlying tuberculous focus from the lymph node or testicles. Initially, it starts as firm, painless, and subcutaneous nodules that gradually enlarge and suppurate, leading to ulcers and sinus tracts with undermined edges and ultimately puckered scars (Fig. 15).

Genital Dermatoses

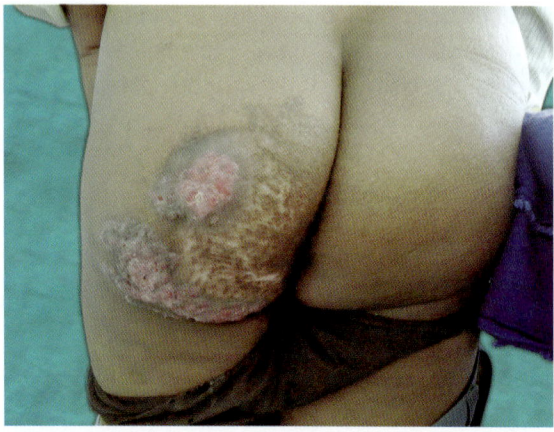

Figure 14: Lupus vulgaris of the gluteal skin who also had matted inguinal lymphadenopathy

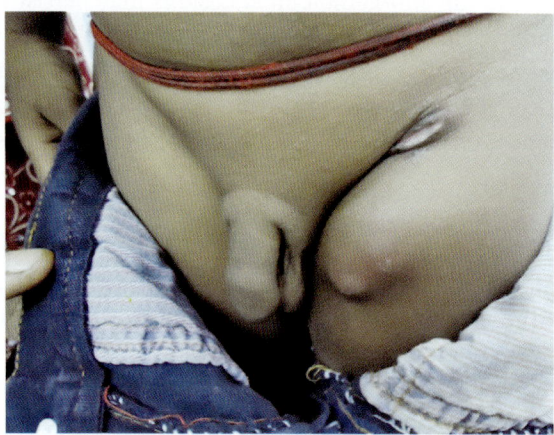

Figure 15: Scrofuloderma in a child

Multiple lesions, failure to respond to treatment should arise suspicion of immunosuppression and multidrug-resistant forms, and HIV infection should be ruled out (Fig. 16).

Genital Infections Other Than Sexually Transmitted Diseases

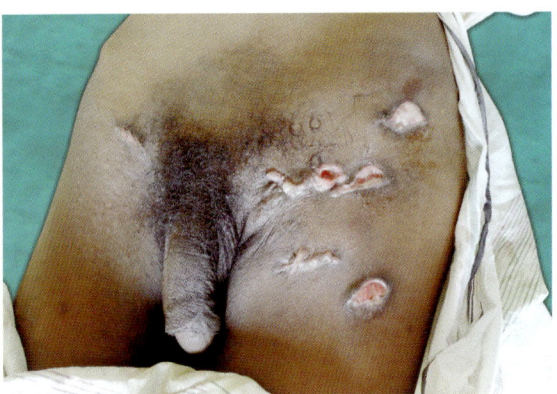

Figure 16: Multiple tuberculous ulcers with discharging sinuses in a HIV positive patient

Systemic involvement should be excluded, whenever there is TB of the ano- genital skin involvement. Early diagnosis and appropriate comprehensive treatment is essential for complete cure.

CUTANEOUS LARVA MIGRANS

Cutaneous larva migrans (CLM) is the most common tropically acquired dermatosis, whose earliest description dates back more than 100 years. CLM clinically presents as itchy, erythematous, serpiginous, and cutaneous eruption caused by accidental percutaneous penetration and subsequent migration of larvae of various nematode parasites. CLM is rare over the genital skin. Like in other sites, it soon goes on for secondary eczematization (Fig. 17 and 18). A good history and astute clinical examination will clinch the diagnosis.

Treatment

Even though CLM is self-limited, the intense pruritus and risk for infection mandate treatment. Once eczematized, low-potency topical steroid cream and oral antihistamines are effective in treating the condition.

Genital Dermatoses

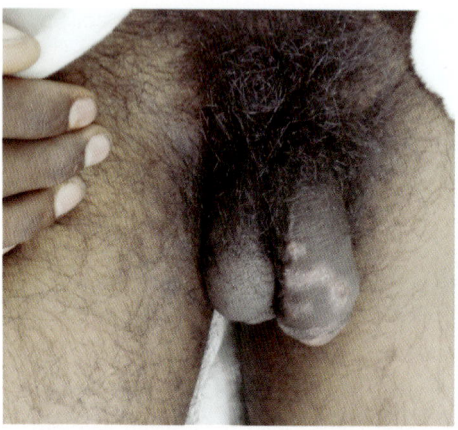

Figure 17: Serpentine rash of cutaneous larva migrans

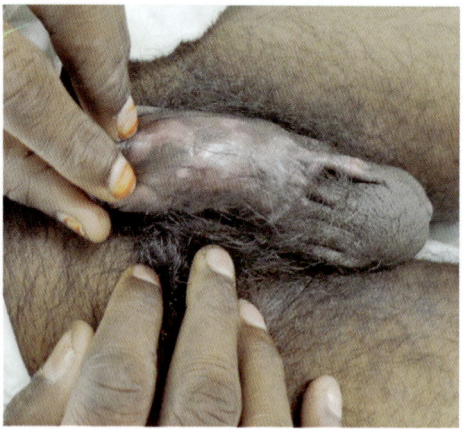

Figure 18: Same as in fig 17 with secondary eczematization

GENERALIZED ERUPTIONS WITH GENITAL INVOLVEMENT

Genital skin can be involved as part of generalized infection. In many patients, an underlying immunosuppression can be

Genital Infections Other Than Sexually Transmitted Diseases

detected. Disseminated baterial and viral infections are common in immunosuppressed individuals (Fig. 19 and 20). Prompt diagnosis and treatment will contain spread of infection.

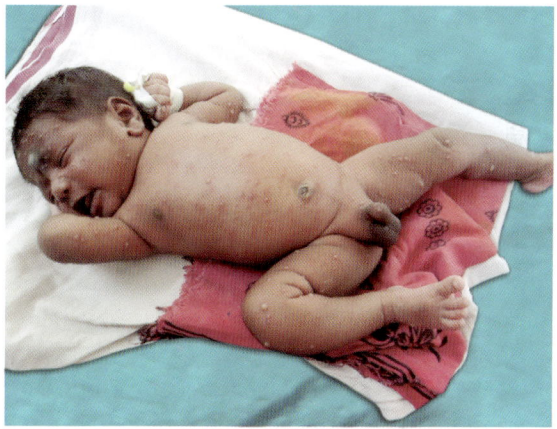

Figure 19: Varicella in an infant with involvement of the genital skin

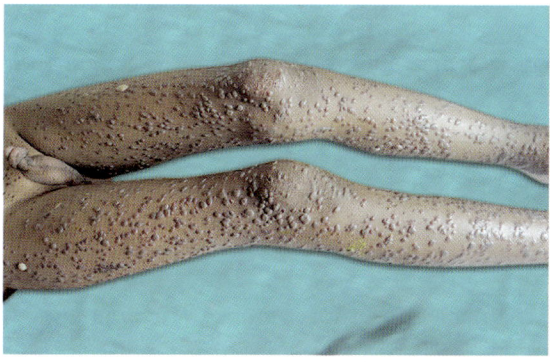

Figure 20: Genital skin involvement in kaposi varicelliform eruption

CHAPTER

8

Bullous Dermatoses

The fragility of blister roof in intertriginous area makes erosions the most common presentation of bullous diseases, which classically appears as blisters elsewhere on skin.

Mucous membrane pemphigoid is a group of chronic inflammatory, autoimmune subepithelial blistering diseases, predominantly affecting mucous membranes and is characterized by linear deposition of immunoglobulin G (IgG), immunoglobulin A (IgA), and complement component C3 along the epithelial basement membrane zone (BMZ). The onset is insidious with few vesicles or bullae on any mucosal surface or less frequently on the skin. The disease most often presents with erosions of oral or conjunctival mucosa, desquamative gingivitis, or conjunctivitis. Genital involvement has been observed in 20% cases. It presents as blisters and erosions on glans penis and prepuce or the labia.

PEMPHIGUS

Pemphigus is a general term for a group of rare autoimmune blistering skin disorders. The two main types of pemphigus are pemphigus vulgaris and pemphigus foliaceus. Each type has subtypes. Additional disorders are sometimes classified as pemphigus including paraneoplastic pemphigus and pemphigus IgA. Autoimmune disorders occur when the body's own immune system mistakenly attacks healthy tissue. The symptoms and severity associated with the various forms of pemphigus vary. All forms of pemphigus are characterized by the development of blistering eruptions on the outer layer of the skin (epidermis). In pemphigus vulgaris, lesions also develop on the mucous membranes, such as those lining the inside of mouth. Mucous membranes are the thin, moist coverings of many of the body's internal surfaces. If left untreated, pemphigus will usually be fatal. The exact cause of pemphigus is unknown. Pemphigus vulgaris presents with cutaneous and oral blisters and erosions. Any stratified squamous mucosal surface (pharyngeal, laryngeal, esophageal, conjunctival, urethral, cervical, or anal) may be affected, particularly in severe disease. Chronic pemphigus may even result in somewhat heaped up, friable, vegetating, papulosquamous plaques in the intertriginous areas (axilla, inframammary folds, and groins) termed pemphigus vegetans.

Pemphigus can be controlled with treatment. If left untreated, serious life-threatening complications, such as the loss of most of the epidermis can occur. Widespread involvement of the skin can also lead to severe infections of the skin, which can potentially spread to the bloodstream (sepsis), or imbalances of fluids or certain minerals (electrolytes) in the body. These imbalances can interfere with various essential chemical processes in the body.

A diagnosis of pemphigus is suspected based upon identification of characteristic findings, a thorough clinical examination, and skin biopsy which reveals the level of acantholysis and immunofluorescence techniques.

Treatment

The mainstay of treatment for pemphigus is the use of high doses of systemic corticosteroids. Other medications that may be used in combination with corticosteroids to treat individuals with pemphigus include drugs that suppress the immune system (immunosuppressive drugs), such as azathioprine, cyclophosphamide, methotrexate, and mycophenolate mofetil; drugs that modify or regulate the immune system (immunomodulatory drugs), such as intravenous immunoglobulin (IVIG), rituxan, dapsone, or antibiotics, such as tetracycline. Combination treatment helps to bring down the overall dose of steroid.

HAILEY-HAILEY DISEASE

Hailey-Hailey disease, also called familial benign chronic pemphigus. It, originally, was described by the Hailey brothers in 1939. Familial benign pemphigus is a chronic autosomal dominant disorder with incomplete penetrance. Approximately, two-third of patients with familial benign pemphigus have a family history of the disorder. An overall defect in keratinocyte adhesion appears to be secondary to a primary defect in a calcium pump protein, calcium-transporting ATPase type 2C member 1 (ATP2C1). Decreased numbers of desmosomes have been implicated in the pathogenesis of benign familial pemphigus. A history of multiple relapses and remissions is characteristic. Precipitating factors include heat, sweating, skin infection, and ultraviolet radiation. The disorder often becomes apparent after puberty, usually by the third or fourth decade, but symptoms can develop at any age. It is characterized clinically by the recurrent eruptions of vesicles and bullae on sides of neck, axilla, groin, genital, and perianal areas. The blister ruptures, leaving an eroded base that exudes serum and forms an impetiginous crust. Mucosal lesions rarely occur, but oral, esophageal, and vaginal involvement has been reported.

Diagnosis of Hailey-Hailey disease is made based upon a thorough clinical evaluation, a detailed patient history, identification of characteristic findings, and microscopic examination (biopsy) of affected skin tissue. A biopsy may reveal abnormal formation of keratin tissue (keratinization) and failure of cell-to-cell adhesion (acantholysis), giving a dilapidated brick wall appearance. Blood tests in individuals with Hailey-Hailey disease will fail to detect antibodies, which rules out autoimmune disorders such as pemphigus.

Treatment

The treatment of Hailey-Hailey disease is directed toward the specific symptoms that are apparent in each individual. Specific therapies depend upon several factors including the extent and severity of the disease and an individual's age and general health.

Individuals with Hailey-Hailey disease are encouraged to avoid "triggers", such as sunburn, sweating, and friction and to keep affected areas dry. For some individuals, sunscreen, loose clothing, moisturizing creams, and avoiding excessive heat may help prevent outbreaks. Cool compresses, dressings, mild corticosteroid creams, and topical antibiotics may be effective in treating mild cases. More serious cases may require systemic antibiotics or stronger corticosteroid creams. Long-term corticosteroid therapy is not recommended because it can further weaken damaged skin over time.

CICATRICIAL PEMPHIGOID (BENIGN MUCOUS MEMBRANE PEMPHIGOID)

Cicatricial pemphigoid (CP) refers to a group of rare, chronic autoimmune blistering diseases, primarily affecting the mucous membranes with resultant scarring. CP is much less common than bullous pemphigoid, but more likely to affect the mucous membrane of the genitalia than does bullous pemphigoid. The age of onset is middle to old age and is more common in women in a ratio of 1.5:1.

It affects the keratinized skin only in about 30% of cases. Because the diagnosis is difficult in the absence of intact blisters on hair-bearing skin, it may be delayed or sometimes missed. It usually starts with irritation, mild blisters, and erosions of mouth, eye, and genitalia. Genital involvement is involved in 50% cases of cicatricial pemphigoid. Men report penile lesions, dysuria, and difficulty retarcting foreskin. Women report pain, pruritus, and dysuria. Morphologically, cicatricial pemphigoid is characterized by painful erosions and scarring. The preceding blisters are often short lived, and the underlying blistering nature of the disease is missed. The mucous membrane erosions may progress rapidly to produce scarring with considerable morbidity. Men may develop meatal stenosis and phimosis, and women may experience urethral stenosis, fusion of the labia, and introitus stenosis. Painful erosions in the mouth are usual. Nasal mucosa, pharynx, and larynx may also be affected, and stridor or dysphagia may result. An ophthalmological examination detects early abnormalities in the eye. Later, more extensive scarring may cause severe adhesions, entropion, and corneal scarring.

Diagnosis

The diagnosis is confirmed by the constellation of ocular, oral, and genital erosions. The diagnosis is confirmed by routine histopathological examination of a blister or erosion. It shows subepidermal blistering, mixed inflammatory infiltrate, and dermal scarring. Diagnosis can be definitely made by immunofluorescence studies. Direct immunofluorescence (DIF) reveals linear deposition on IgG, IgA, and C3 at the BMZ.

Treatment

The goals of treatment for CP are to reduce symptoms (pain) and to induce a degree of remission to minimize scarring.

Systemic steroids may be helpful for skin disease but less helpful for mucosal lesions. Steroid sparing drugs (dapsone, cyclophosphamide, and azathioprine) may be used. More recently, IVIG has shown promise in the treatment of the disease. Genital lesions may be improved by potent topical steroids. Surgery and dilatation may be needed to alleviate scarring when the skin disease is controlled.

ERYTHEMA MULTIFORME

Erythema multiforme (EM) is an acute, self-limiting, type IV hypersensitivity reaction of the skin and mucous membranes described by Hebra in 1866. It is characterized by symmetrically distributed skin lesions, located primarily on the extremities, and by a tendency for recurrences, affecting mostly children and young adults. The cause is unknown, but EM frequently occurs in association with herpes simplex virus (HSV), suggesting an immunologic process initiated by the virus. In half of the cases, the triggering agents appear to be medications, including anticonvulsants, sulfonamides, nonsteroidal anti-inflammatory drugs (NSAIDs), and other antibiotics.

Erythema multiforme is characterized by target or iris lesions of the skin. It may be episodic or recurrent with great variability in the interval between episodes. Previously, the condition was thought to be part of a clinical spectrum of disease that also included two more severe forms, Stevens-Johnson syndrome (SJS), and toxic epidermal necrolysis (TEN). Nonetheless, there is increasing evidence that the latter two are distinct from EM, due to their contrasting clinical presentations and potential causes.

Erythema multiforme is a self-limited eruption that usually has mild or no prodromal symptoms. Patients may experience itching and burning at the site of the eruption. The individual lesions begin acutely as numerous sharply-demarcated red or pink macules that then become papular. The papules may enlarge gradually into plaques several centimeters in diameter. The central portion of the papules or plaques gradually becomes dark red, brown, dusky or, purpuric. Crusting or blistering sometimes occurs in the center of the lesions. The characteristic "target" or "iris" lesion has a regular round shape and three concentric zones: a central dusky or darker red area, a paler pink or edematous zone, and a peripheral red ring. Some target lesions have only two zones, the dusky or darker red center and a pink or lighter red border. The skin lesions of EM usually appear symmetrically on the distal extremities and progress proximally. Palms and soles also may be involved. Mucosal lesions may occur.

Treatment

Mild cases of EM do not require treatment. Oral antihistamines and topical steroids may be used to provide symptom relief. In patients with coexisting or recent HSV infection, early treatment with oral acyclovir may lessen the number and duration of cutaneous lesions. Prednisone may be used in patients with many lesions at dosages of 40–80 mg per day for 1–2 weeks, then tapered rapidly.

STEVENS-JOHNSON SYNDROME

Stevens-Johnson syndrome and toxic epidermal necrolysis are the acute emergencies in dermatology practice. SJS and TEN involve less than 10% and more than 30% of the body surface area, respectively. The third condition named as SJS-TEN overlap falls in-between SJS and TEN. Patient may initially present with SJS, which subsequently evolves into TEN or SJS-TEN overlap. The exact mechanism of SJS and TEN still remains largely unknown. Immunological mechanisms, reactive drug metabolites or interactions between these two are proposed.

Initial symptoms of TEN and SJS can be unspecific and include symptoms such as fever, stinging eyes, and discomfort upon swallowing. Typically, these symptoms precede cutaneous manifestations by a few days. Early sites of cutaneous involvement are the presternal region of the trunk and the face, but also the palms and soles. Involvement of the buccal, genital, and/or ocular mucosa occurs in more than 90% of patients, and in some cases the respiratory and gastrointestinal tracts are also affected. Clinical signs initially include areas of erythematous and livid macules on the skin on which a positive Nikolsky's sign can be elicited. Soon these develop erosions which may be difficult to treat, if infected (Figs 1 to 4). Mucosal involvement develops shortly before or simultaneously with skin signs in almost all cases.

Treatment

Management in the acute stage involves sequentially evaluating the severity and prognosis of disease, prompt identification and withdrawal of the culprit drugs, and rapidly initiating supportive care in an appropriate setting. Systemic steroids and high-dose IVIG can be given assessing the risk benefit ratio.

FIXED DRUG ERUPTION

Fixed drug eruption (FDE) always recurs at the same sites on re-exposure to the drug or agent. Antibiotics are the most common

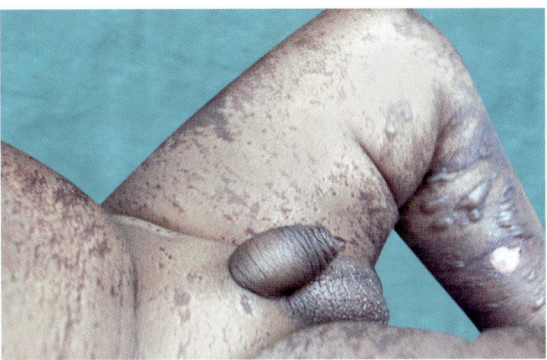

Figure 1: Erythematous and livid macules on the pubic and genital skin in a child with stevens-johnson syndrome

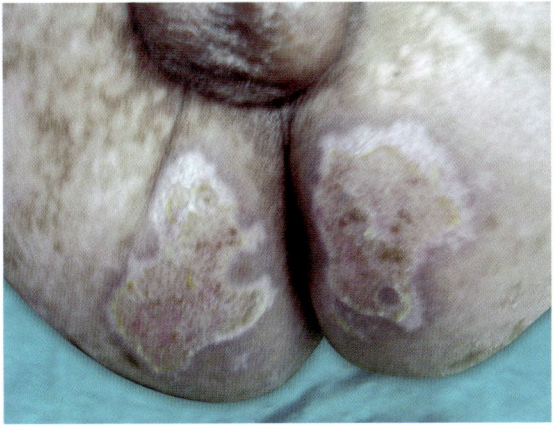

Figure 2: Same child with stevens-johnson syndrome as in fig 1 developing large area of erosion

cause, especially sulfonamides and tetracyclines, but many other drugs have been reported including terbinafine and NSAIDs. The mechanism of this reaction involves immune cells (lymphocytes) called memory CD8+ T cells that remain in a fixed area of skin.

The most common sites are the lips, genital area, hands, and feet. On the first occasion, it begins 1–2 weeks after drug exposure as one or more sharply-defined red swollen lesions that may develop a

Genital Dermatoses

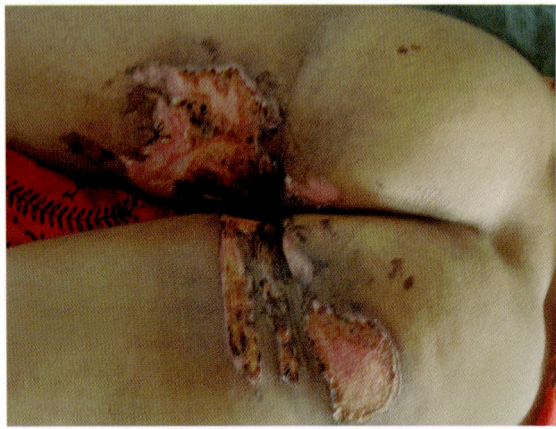

Figure 3: Skin with positive Nikolsky's sign in toxic epidermal necrolysis

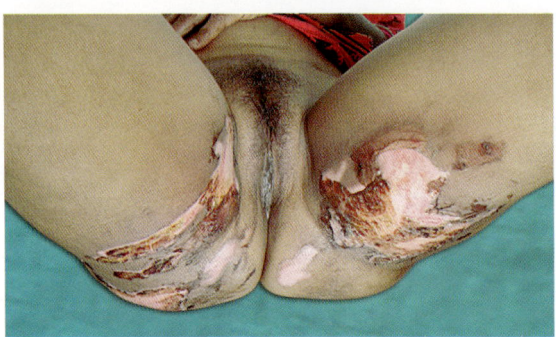

Figure 4: Toxic epidermal necrolysis showing desquamation of the skin in a patient who had severe genital mucosal involvement

central clear blister. It settles over several days, leaving round to oval shaped areas of pigmentation (Fig. 5).

With every further exposure, the reaction appears more quickly (i.e., within 24 hours), is more inflamed, and the residual pigmentation darkens. The severity of reactions in FDE may increase after repeated exposures to the drug and very rarely progress to a clinical state, so called generalized bullous FDE. Generalized bullous FDE with its characteristic multiple large, purplish-livid patches, at

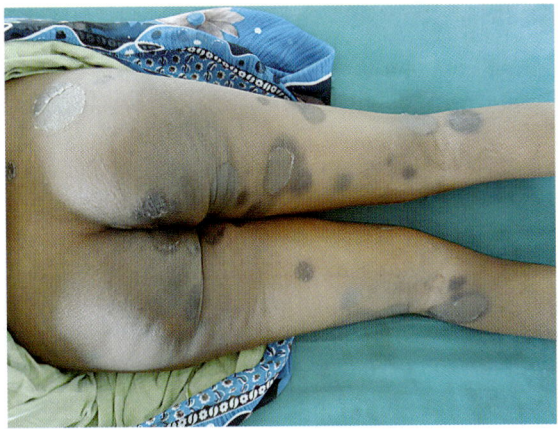

Figure 5: Fucid drug eruption of the gluteal skin. This lady also had involvement of the skin over labia

times with flaccid blisters, may be clinically misdiagnosed as SJS or TEN. In generalized bullous FDE, the disease onset is within hours after the drug exposure. A diagnostic hallmark is the reappearance of the lesions over the previously affected sites, when the offending drug is reused.

Histopathological differentiation of generalized bullous FDE from SJS and TEN may be challenging. Epidermal changes varying from a few scattered necrotic keratinocytes to full thickness epidermal necrosis cannot be distinguished in all three conditions. In FDE, a mixed inflammatory infiltrate containing not only lymphocytes but also neutrophils and eosinophils is present around both the superficial and deep plexus. In SJS and TEN, the infiltrate is mainly lymphohistiocytic and tends to be located around the superficial plexus.

Treatment

Treatment is aimed at identifying and stopping the offending drug. In mild cases, the application of topical steroid is sufficient. Systemic steroids are warranted in severe cases. The residual pigmentation is difficult to treat and may take several years for complete clearance.

LINEAR IMMUNOGLOBULIN A DERMATOSIS

Linear immunoglobulin A dermatosis (LAD) is an autoimmune subepidermal vesiculobullous disease that may be idiopathic or drug induced, and DR3 has been reported. Vancomycin is the most common drug incriminated, while others include captopril, penicillin, ceftriaxone, sulfonamides, furosemide, lithium, phenytoin, carbamazepine, glibenclamide, atorvastatin, and NSAIDs.

Antibody deposition leads to complement activation and neutrophil chemotaxis, which results in loss of adhesion at the dermal-epidermal junction and blister formation. IgA autoantibodies from LAD sera react with antigens of 97 and 120 kDa, both of which are fragments of the extracellular domain of bullous pemphigoid antigen 180 (type XVII collagen). Antibodies have also been found to act against bullous pemphigoid antigen 230 and collagen VII rarely.

Clinical Features

Linear immunoglobulin A dermatosis have a bimodal age of onset: childhood type [originally known as chronic bullous disease of childhood (CBDC)] appearing before the age of 5 and the adult linear IgA disease appearing after the age of 40 years with a slight female predilection. Cutaneous lesions in LAD are heterogeneous and may mimic other bullous diseases. In children, the onset is usually acute and presents as papules, urticarial plaques, and polycyclic lesions with blisters situated mainly on the face, abdomen, and perineum (Fig. 6). Mucosal involvement with scarring may occur. Children may present with genital and perioral blisters, suggesting the possibility of sexual abuse. The adult variant is characterized by vesicles and bullae occurring less symmetrically than those seen in dermatitis herpetiformis, but may be distributed in similar locations. The tendency for new blisters to arise in a ring around an old one is called the "string of beads" sign which is usually present in children.

Diagnosis

Histologically, LAD shows subepidermal blisters with an infiltrate, primarily consisting of neutrophils. DIF of perilesional skin usually

Bullous Dermatoses

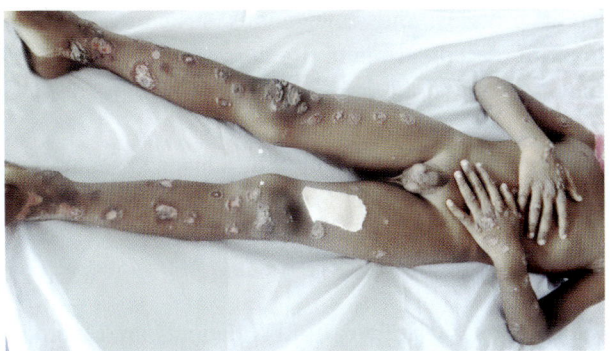

Figure 6: Genital skin involvement of Linear IgA dermatoses

shows deposition of IgA along the BMZ in a homogeneous linear pattern. Granular linear deposition at the BMZ along with IgG and C3 deposition are also found rarely. The differential diagnosis of this condition includes other subepidermal bullous disorders like dermatitis herpetiformis, epidermolysis bullosa acquisita, bullous pemphigoid, and bullous systemic lupus erythematosus.

Treatment

Dapsone is the drug of choice for patients with LAD. The response is rapid and most lesions resolve within 48-72 hours as seen in our case also. Flucloxacillin and sulfamethoxypyridazine have also been tried in few cases as second line treatment with good results. Tetracycline, erythromycin, niacinamide, colchicines, systemic corticosteroids, mycophenolate mofetil, methotrexate, cyclosporine, azathioprine, interferon-α, thalidomide, and IVIG are the other successful modes of therapy.

EPIDERMOLYSIS BULLOSA ACQUISITA

Epidermolysis bullosa acquisita (EBA) is a rare, autoimmune subepidermal blistering skin condition characterized by abnormal immunoglobulins against a predominant component of the basement membrane, collagen VII. The epidermal BMZ consists of different proteins and collagenous structures that facilitate attachment of the epidermis to the dermis. Collagen VII has been identified as the major component of anchoring fibrils and is involved in a series of complex interactions. Presence of abnormal autoantibodies leads to separation of the dermal-epidermal junction and formation of subepidermal blisters.

Clinical Features

The cutaneous manifestations in EBA patients are heterogeneous. However, EBA patients can be classified into two major clinical subtypes: noninflammatory (classical or mechanobullous) and inflammatory, which is characterized by cutaneous inflammation resembling bullous pemphigoid, LAD, mucous membrane pemphigoid or Brunsting-Perry pemphigoid. The clinical presentation of an individual EBA patient may change during the course of the disease or the same patients may present with two different forms, simultaneously. On the genitals, painful erosions are typical, and scarring may lead to phimosis in uncircumcised men and alteration of normal vulval architecture and introital stenosis in women. Scarring of the conjunctiva, larynx, and esophagus also occurs. EBA has been known to be associated with internal malignancies (e.g., lung, bowel, or hematological). Junctional and dystrophic EB can rarely involve the genital mucosa (Fig. 7).

Diagnosis

Histopathological findings include subepidermal blistering with a mixed inflammatory cell infiltrate, low in eosinophils, and minimal blood vessel wall thickening. DIF demonstrates linear deposits of IgG and/or C3 at the dermal-epidermal junction. Bullous pemphigoid has a similar immunofluorescence appearance, but can be distinguished from EBA by salt skin splitting where the dermal-epidermal junction is separated through the lamina lucida zone and the bullous pemphigoid antigen is placed on the epidermal side, whereas EBA antigens are found on the dermal side.

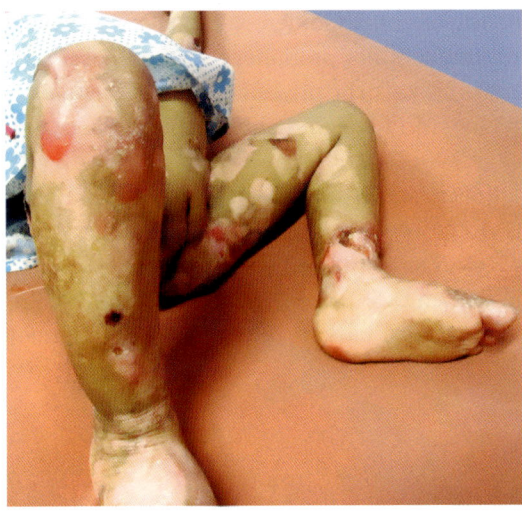

Figure 7: Involvement of skin over the inner thigh in a child with epidermolysis bullosa acquisita

Treatment

Treatment is difficult, and the course of EBA is prolonged. It may be unresponsive to steroids or to immunosuppressive agents. Supportive care is essential, especially, if the disease is widespread, and careful attention to the secondary infection on genitalia may help to minimize scarring.

PEMPHIGOID GESTATIONIS (HERPES GESTATIONIS)

Pemphigoid gestationis (PG) or herpes gestationis is a rare, autoimmune subepidermal blistering disorder associated with pregnancy, with autoantibodies targeting the hemidesmosomal proteins BP180 and less commonly BP230. The condition typically develops during the second or third trimester of pregnancy, but has been rarely reported in the first trimester and postpartum period. Recurrence of the skin lesions in subsequent pregnancies and postpartum flare-up may indicate the persistence of circulating autoantibodies. It starts as intensely pruritic, erythematous annular urticarial plaques on which blisters develop. The lesions are described more frequently on the abdomen, with extension to flexural areas. Vulvar involvement is not prominent, and mucosal involvement is mild. Fetal risks may also be present in PG and include miscarriages, prematurity, low birth weight babies, and transient erythema and blistering.

Histopathology shows subepidermal bulla containing numerous eosinophils. The essential component for the diagnosis of PG is the finding of C3 with or without IgG in a linear band along the BMZ of perilesional skin on DIF.

Systemic corticosteroids are the mainstay of treatment.

CHAPTER

9

Inflammatory Lesions of the Genitalia

LICHEN SCLEROSUS ET ATROPHICUS

Lichen sclerosus et atrophicus (LSA) is a rare, inflammatory disease of unknown etiology. Hallopeau is credited with the first clinical description of LSA in 1887 and Darrier first reported histopathological changes in 1892. Disease predominates in females and may occur at any age. However, the maximum incidence occurs between the 5th and 6th decades of life, perimenopausal group, and another peak in girls between the ages 8 and 13 years, prepubertal group. In both the sexes, anogenital involvement is common. Balanitis xerotica obliterans is now viewed as a synonymous term, describing LSA of the penis, and "kraurosis vulvae" is now recognized as LSA of the vulva. Extragenital involvement is associated with classic genital LSA in 15-20% of cases.

Etiology

Although the exact cause is unknown, lichen sclerosus (LS) is a disease of multifactorial etiology. Associated factors include:
- Genetic predisposition
- Epigenetic factors
- Autoimmune diseases
- Hormonal influences
- Infectious triggers
- A stressed immune system.

Lichen sclerosus may be more common in some families and can often be triggered by trauma, hormonal changes, infection, and surgery. Patients with LS have a higher risk of developing other autoimmune disorders. Associated autoimmune disorders may include thyroid disease, anemia, diabetes, alopecia areata, and vitiligo.

Clinical Features

In females, the typical lesions are porcelain-white papules and plaques, often associated with areas of ecchymosis. The characteristic sites are the interlabial sulci, labia minora, clitoral hood, clitoris, perineal body, and perineum (Figs 1 to 8). Genital mucosal involvement does not occur, the vagina and cervix always being spared [which is in contrast to lichen planus (LP)], although there may be involvement at the mucocutaneous junctions (the vestibule), which may result in introital narrowing, also referred to as "keyhole or hourglass." Perianal lesions occur in women in 30% of cases. There may be extension to the buttocks and genitocrural folds. LS can koebnerize and may first arise in an episiotomy scar.

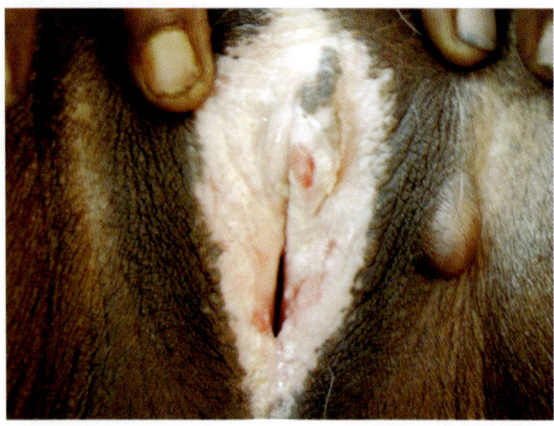

Figure 1: Porcelain-white sclerotic plaques of lichen sclerosus et atrophicus involving the labia and clitoris

Itch is the main symptom, but pain may be a consequence of erosions or fissures. However, LS may also be entirely asymptomatic and an incidental finding on examination. Dyspareunia occurs in the presence of erosions, fissures, or introital narrowing.

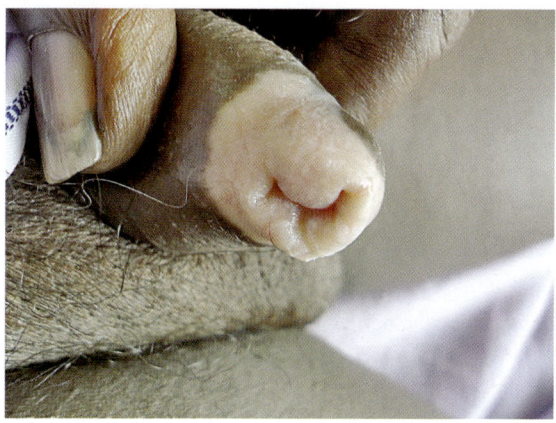

Figure 2: Lichen sclerosus et atrophicus of the penile skin, note the shiny sclerosed area

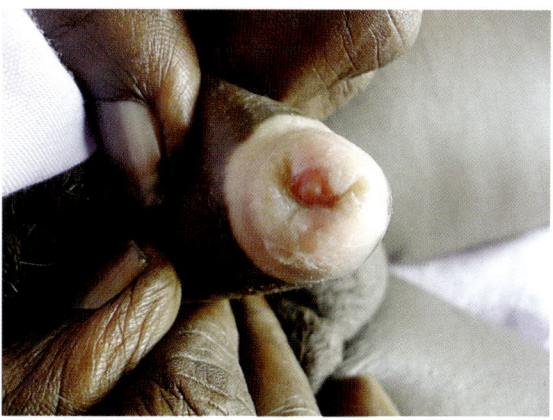

Figure 3: Lichen sclerosus et atrophicus almost stenosing the meatus

Genital Dermatoses

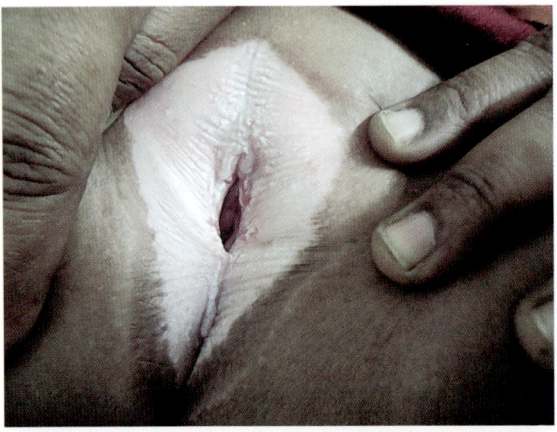

Figure 4: Lichen sclerosus et atrophicus over pre-existing vitiligo showing narrowing of the introitus

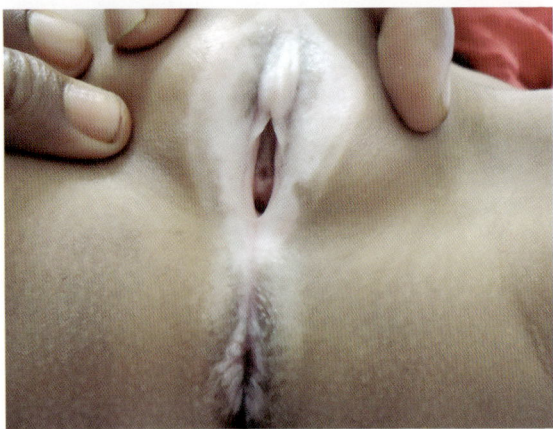

Figure 5: Vitiligo with Lichen sclerosus et atrophicus figure of 8 distributions

In males, the common sites of involvement of LS in adult men are the prepuce, coronal sulcus, and glans penis, and more rarely lesions may be found on the shaft of the penis. The presenting complaint is usually tightening of the foreskin, which may lead to phimosis. This in turn results in erectile dysfunction and painful erections. Perianal disease is rarely, if ever, seen in male patients. The perimeatal

Inflammatory Lesions of the Genitalia

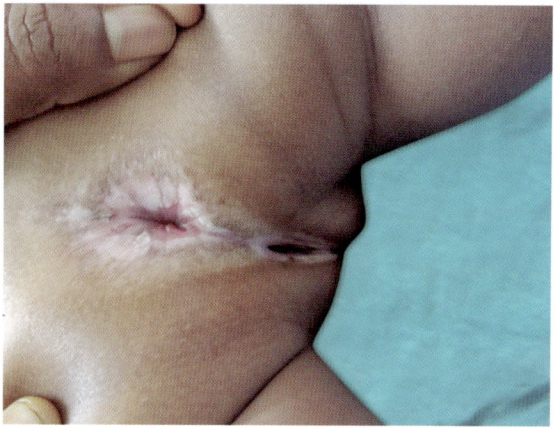

Figure 6: Same as in figure 5 showing the perianal involvement

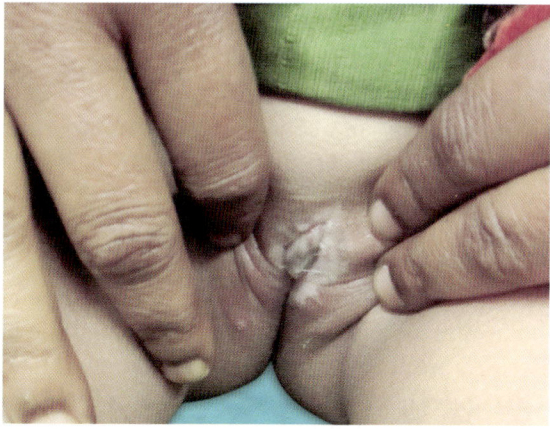

Figure 7: Lichen sclerosus et atrophicus in a three year old child note the sclerosis and superficial fissure

area may be involved and postinflammatory scarring may lead to stenosis and obstruction. There may also be more proximal urethral involvement, although this usually starts at the meatus. These complications may require a multidisciplinary approach with input from both a dermatologist and urologist.

Genital Dermatoses

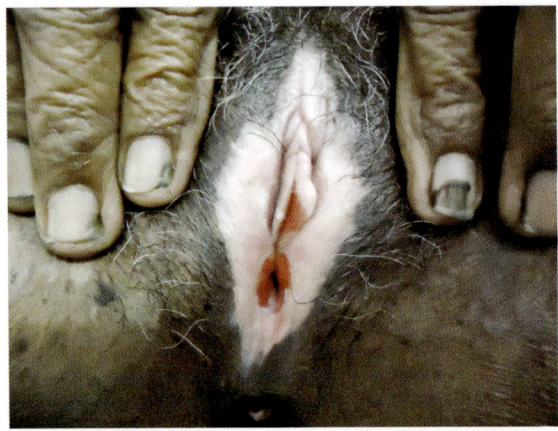

Figure 8: Vitiligo with lichen sclerosus et atrophicus showing erosion

Histopathology

Histologically, LSA has a characteristic pattern. Histologically well-developed lesion of LSA is characterized by marked orthohyperkeratosis, keratotic plugging of the hair follicles and dermal appendages, atrophy of stratum malpighi with flattening, and loss of rete ridges. The basal layer shows liquefactive degeneration. Beneath the epidermis, there is broad zone of pronounced edema and homogenization of the collagen. Within this zone, collagen fibers are swollen, homogenous, and contain very few nuclei. The blood and lymphatic vessels are dilated, and there may be areas of hemorrhage. Edema in the upper part of the dermis may be enough to result in clinically apparent vesiculation. The lower dermis is characterized by the presence of dense lymphocytic infiltrate in the mid dermis, which drifts from its subepidermal position to mid dermis as the lesion develops on account of the edema and homogenization of collagen in the upper dermis.

Prognosis

Lichen sclerosus is a chronic condition, but there may be waxing and waning of signs and symptoms. Anogenital LS involutes by menarche in approximately two thirds of prepubertal cases, the remaining one third have persistent atrophy. After puberty, resolution of lesions is unlikely. Premalignant changes may occur, with a 4–5% risk of developing squamous cell carcinoma (SCC) in vulval LS. There is an increased incidence of genitourinary infections.

Differential Diagnosis

Anogenital LS in females closely mimics vitiligo, genital LP, lichen simplex chronicus, and extra mammary Paget's disease. In males, anogenital LS needs to be differentiated from balanoposthitis, idiopathic phimosis, and erosive LP.

Treatment

The aims of managing LS are to treat the symptoms of itching, burning, and pain; heal the cutaneous lesions; reduce further scarring; and to prevent or detect malignant changes. Genital LS may respond to potent topical corticosteroids, although the patient should be warned that the clinical appearance does not always reverse even if symptoms are relieved. The calcineurin inhibitors (i.e., tacrolimus and, pimecrolimus) have been found to help some patients, especially with genital LS, but they do not work as fast or as effectively as potent topical corticosteroids. Circumcision may benefit male LS and the phimosis that may accompany it. Vulvar surgery is not recommended unless an associated malignancy is present.

LICHEN PLANUS

Lichen planus is an inflammatory papulosquamous dermatosis which can affect the skin, nails and all mucous membranes, including the genitalia. The initial description was given by Hebra and later, Eramus Wilson (1869) had given it the name.

The etiology is largely unknown but thought to involve an autoimmune mechanism of activated T-cells directed against basal keratinocytes. It is associated with the DR1 human leukocyte antigen (HLA) class II antigen. It can also be drug induced with

Genital Dermatoses

β-blockers, NSAIDs, angiotensin-converting enzyme (ACE) inhibitors, lithium, methyldopa, quinine, carbamazepine, and penicillamine all—being linked to the condition.

Clinical Features

In females, it occurs in the peri and postmenopausal period. This presents with vulval soreness, burning, pruritis, dyspareunia, postcoital bleeding, persistent and copious vaginal discharge, dysuria or difficulty in urinating. Often these symptoms are incorrectly attributed to persistent candidiasis.

Three types of LP can affect the vulva or vagina (Figs. 9 to 12):

1. Papulosquamous: Small pruritic papules; involves keratinized and perianal skin.
2. Hypertrophic: Rarest form with appearances similar to vulval SCC; hypertrophic and rough lesions on perineum and perianal area.
3. Erosive (as in our case): Glassy and brightly erythematous erosions with white striae or a white border (Wickham's striae); architectural destruction with loss of the labia minora and clitoris

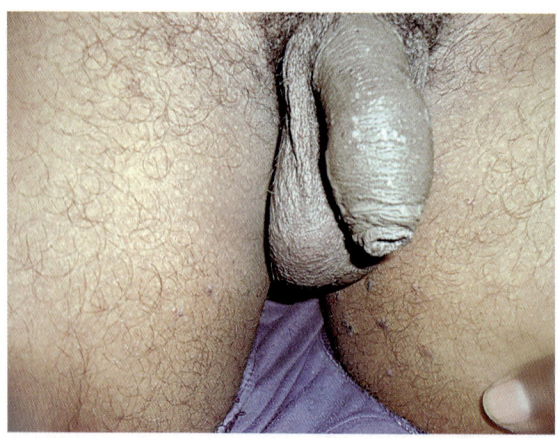

Figure 9: Violaceous papules over upper medial aspect of thigh and shaft of penis

and narrowing of the introitus. The epithelium is denuded, leading to contact bleeding, discharge, and vaginal adhesions. Care must be taken when obtaining biopsies; this is because, if only areas of erosion are sampled, features associated with LP will

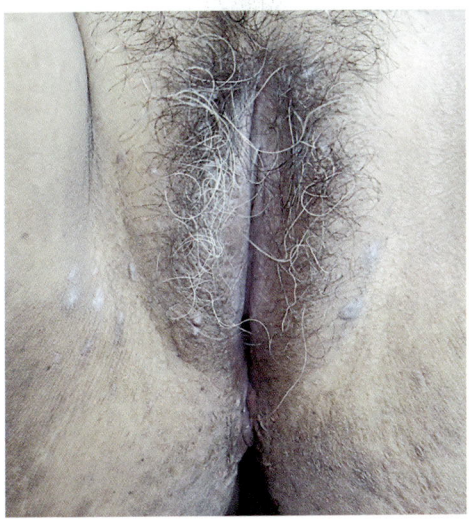

Figure 10: Lichen Planus of genital skin

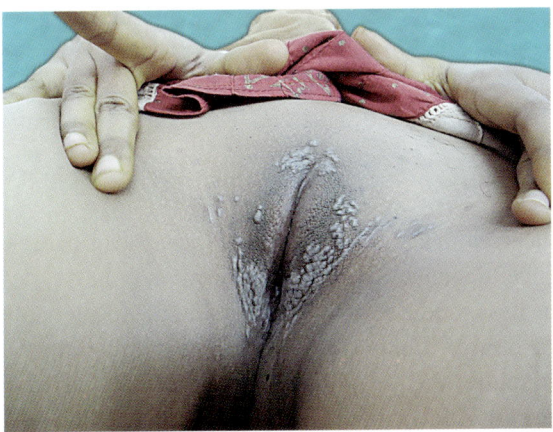

Figure 11: Lichen planus of the genital area exhibiting Koebner's phenomenon

Genital Dermatoses

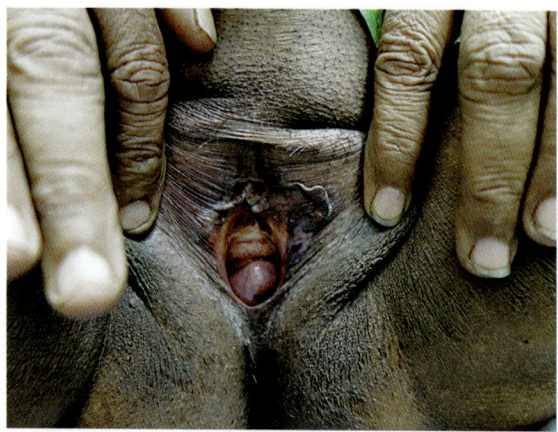

Figure 12: Erosive lichen planus, note the violaceuos border

not be found, but instead those of desquamative inflammatory vaginitis—acute and chronic inflammation involving the mucosa and submucosa.

In 25% of men with cutaneous LP, the genitalia are involved. The lesions involve the shaft, glans penis, prepuce, or scrotum. Annular LP is the most common morphology seen in the male genitalia.

The combination of vulvovaginal LP and desquamative gingivitis is termed as vulvovaginal-gingival syndrome. A similar condition in males, "peno-gingival LP" is rare. SCC is a rare complication.

Histopathology

Histological features of LP are irregular acanthosis of the epidermis, liquefactive degeneration of the basal cell layer, degenerative keratinocytes (colloid or civatte bodies) in the lower epidermis, and band-like dermal infiltrate of lymphocytes in the upper epidermis. The epithelium may be absent with areas of hyperkeratosis. DIF study reveals globular deposits of immunoglobulin M (IgM) and complement mixed with apoptotic keratinocytes.

Treatment

Potent topical corticosteroids are most effective for mucosal LP. Topical calcineurin inhibitors like cyclosporine, tacrolimus, and pimecrolimus have been used. Oral medications include corticosteroids, retinoids, and cyclosporin.

HIDRADENITIS SUPPURATIVA

Hidradenitis suppurativa (HS), first described in 1839 by Velpeau, is a chronic disease, manifested by recurrent abscesses, sinus tracts, and scarring. This disease typically affects the genitofemoral area in women or axillae in both sexes. It is also known as Verneuil's disease or acne inversa. It is a member of the follicular occlusion tetrad along with acne conglobata, dissecting cellulitis of the scalp, and pilonidal sinus.

Etiology and Pathogenesis

The etiology of HS is still under debate. While several studies have failed to demonstrate human lymphocyte antigens associations, others have suggested an autosomal dominant mode of inheritance. Otherwise, a hyperandrogenism, obesity via occlusion and maceration, heat, humidity and friction from clothing, smoking, lithium, chemical irritants, and oral contraceptives may be associated with HS, possibly as triggering factors. Several disease entities have been reported as being associated with HS including Crohn's disease, Dowling-Degos disease (acquired reticulate pigmented macules in the flexures), and arthropathy.

Little is known about its cause to date, but it is thought that the initial event is follicular hyperkeratosis with occlusion of the follicle. Dilatation of the follicle is followed by rupture and spillage of contents into the surrounding dermis. This induces a chemotactic response with a resultant inflammatory cell infiltrate. The apocrine glands are secondarily involved, and secondary infection may also occur.

Clinical Features

Hidradenitis suppurativa is more common in women, with a ratio of three females to each male affected. Onset is most common from childhood to middle age with a peak during puberty.

The disease is essentially limited to areas of the skin that are rich in terminal hair follicles and apocrine glands such as the axilla, the anogenital area, and the mammary glands.

Clinically, it is characterized by recurring pustules, inflammatory nodules, abscesses, draining sinus formation, fibrosis, secondary lymphedema, and double-ended pseudo-comedone (Figs 13 to 15). HS is not acne; closed comedones are not seen, since the deep part of the follicle appears to be involved but not its superficial compartment, as seen with acne affecting convex skin surfaces. HS inflammatory lesions are initially transient, but gradually become intransigent and associated with significant scarring.

The severity of HS can be varied ranging from mild (stage 1), with small nodules without abscess or sinus tract formation; to moderate (stage 2), where abscesses and sinuses occur causing discomfort and problems with drainage but may variably respond to medical treatment options; to severe (stage 3), with extensive-scarring, multiple sinuses, and fistula formation. This stage usually requires

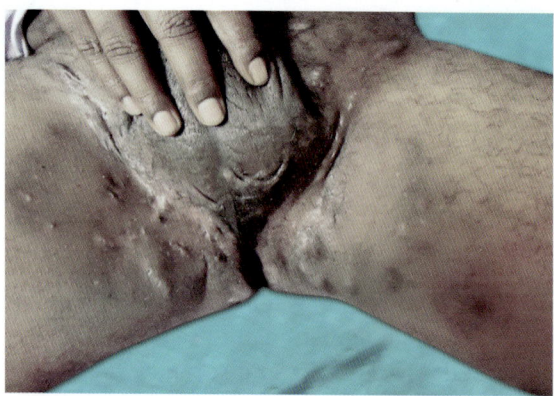

Figure 13: Multiple nodules with scarring and sinuses over pubic region, perianal, and groin

Inflammatory Lesions of the Genitalia

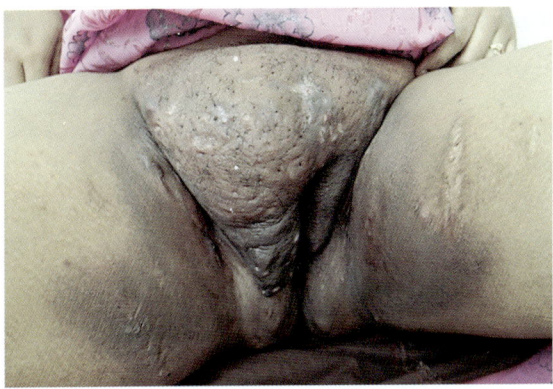

Figure 14: Hidradenitis suppurativa in woman showing multiple scars

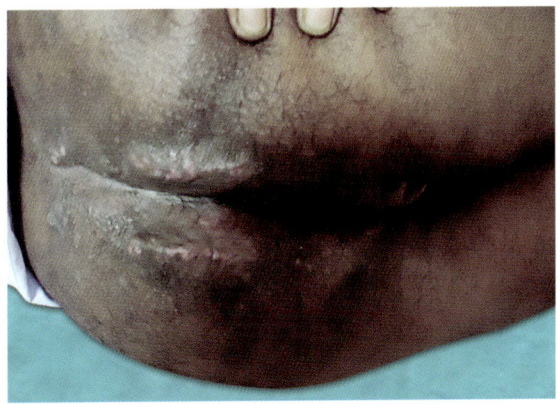

Figure 15: Nodules and scarring over gluteal and perianal region, note the linear scar of surgery

definitive surgical management, after initial medical management to control the sinuses successfully.

Bacterial infection of the structurally abnormal areas is felt to be a secondary event rather than the initial factor and contributes to the destructive nature and extension of the lesions. *S. aureus* and coagulase-negative *Staphylococci* are commonly found along with others including *Peptostreptococcus* species and *Propionibacterium acnes*.

Complications

Potential complications include dermal contraction, local or disseminated infection, lymphedema caused by lymphatic injury from inflammation and scarring, and rectal or urethral fistulas. Reports of SCC following chronic lesions of HS have been described.

Differential Diagnosis

The differential diagnosis includes carbuncles, lymphadenitis, and infected Bartholin's or sebaceous cysts. Differential diagnosis of discharging sinuses will include: tuberculous scrofuloderma, atypical mycobacterial infections, actinomycosis, sporotrichosis, botryomycosis, and nocardiosis.

Treatment

Much of the medical management centers around systemic and/or topical antibacterial agents and general skin-care measures (avoidance of irritation of the affected area, weight loss, and stopping smoking).

Topical clindamycin, oral clindamycin, tetracycline, minocycline, and erythromycin are commonly used for mild to moderate HS. However, there are concerns about long-term monotherapy and development of resistance.

Anti-androgen treatments, such as cyproterone acetate used with ethinylestradiol and finasteride (a 5-α-reductase inhibitor) can be useful treatment options, although the link between HS and androgens is still controversial.

Patients treated with antitumor necrosis factor-α treatments such as infliximab and etanercept have also shown improvement and this may be due to underlying immune mechanisms.

In addition, oral retinoids, such as acitretin and etretinate have been shown to have some success in the treatment of HS.

Wide surgical excision, with margins well beyond the clinical borders of activity, remains the most definitive surgical therapy.

More limited surgical intervention, consisting of unroofing abscesses and sinus tracts, with vigorous curettage of the base, and secondary-intention healing can be valuable in some cases. Laser treatment with carbon dioxide is an alternative in mild to moderate cases.

BEHCET'S DISEASE

Behcet's disease is a multisystem inflammatory disorder characterized by recurrent oral ulcers, genital ulcers, and ocular inflammation, and which frequently involves the joints, skin, central nervous system (CNS), and gastrointestinal tract. Classified as a systemic vasculitis, it can involve both the arteries and veins of almost any organ.

Etiology and Pathogenesis

The genetic locus most widely studied in Behcet's disease is the HLA complex on chromosome 6p21. Disease susceptibility has consistently been associated with polymorphisms in the HLA-B gene, particularly HLA-B*51. Although it is clear that there is a significant genetic component to susceptibility to Behcet's disease, environmental factors also play a role. The most plausible environmental trigger is an infectious agent, and evidence of ongoing or previous infection with a variety of viral agents has been sought. These include HSV-1, the hepatitis viruses, and parvovirus B19.

Potential bacterial triggers include mycobacteria, *Borrelia burgdorferi, Helicobacter pylori,* and a variety of streptococcal antigens.

Alternatively, Behcet's disease may be primarily autoimmune in origin. This does not exclude an infective trigger, which could operate through molecular mimicry or some other mechanism, but implies that the disease is perpetuated by an abnormal immune response to an autoantigen in the absence of ongoing infection. A number of factors mitigate against a classic autoimmune origin, including the lack of association with other autoimmune diseases, the lack of association with the autoimmune HLA haplotype (HLA-

A1-B8-DR3), the lack of a female preponderance, and the absence of organ-nonspecific autoantibodies, such as antinuclear antibodies. There is, however, no doubt that an inflammatory response to several autoantigens is found in Behcet's disease. Antiendothelial antibodies, for example, are a frequent but nonspecific finding.

Pathology

The common histopathological lesion underlying the clinical manifestations of Behcet's disease is vasculitis, involving particularly the venules. Lesions are characterized by perivascular lymphocytic and monocytic cellular infiltration, with or without fibrin deposition in the vessel wall and surrounding tissue necrosis. Significant neutrophil infiltration is also seen, particularly in early lesions including those of the pathergy reaction.

Clinical Features

Recurrent aphthous ulceration is the characteristic feature of Behcet's disease. Oral ulcers are usually the earliest sign of disease and may precede the onset of systemic symptoms by many years. Lesions may occur singly or in crops, and subside without scarring. The most common sites of oral ulceration are the tongue, lips, and gingival and buccal mucosa, although involvement of the palate, pharynx, and tonsil can also occur. Oral ulcers may be classified into minor ulcers (diameter 10 mm, shallow, surrounded by an erythematous halo and healing without scarring), major ulcers (morphologically similar but larger, more painful, and more persistent, and which may leave a scar on healing), and herpetiform ulcers. Genital ulcers occur in 72–94% of cases and are morphologically similar to oral ulcers but frequently heal by scarring (Figs 16 and 17). In males, they most commonly occur on the scrotum, and penile lesions are uncommon. Epididymitis is also common, but urethritis is not a feature of Behcet's disease, which may be useful in distinguishing it from Reiter's syndrome. In females, ulcers occur on the vulva, vagina, and cervix, and may cause dyspareunia. Groin, perianal, and perineal ulcers occur in both sexes.

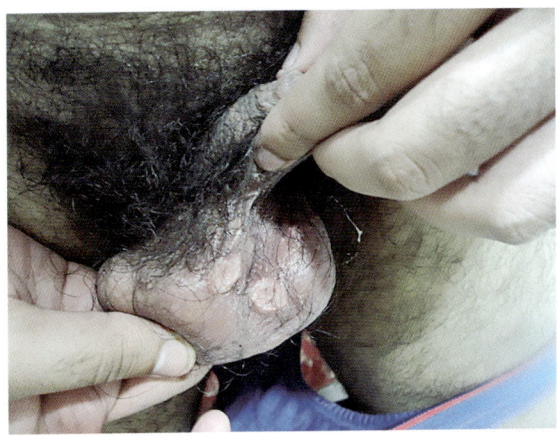

Figure 16: Behcet disease's Multiple painful ulcers with sloping edges and necrotic base seen over scrotum

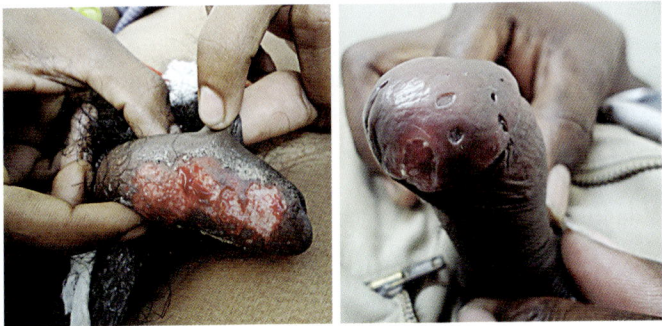

Figure 17: Penile ulcer, an uncommon site in Behcets's disease

Ocular involvement is reported in 30-70% of patients with Behcet's disease. Chronic, relapsing bilateral uveitis involving both the anterior and posterior uveal tracts is a significant cause of morbidity. Anterior uveitis with hypopyon, in which the inflammatory exudate forms a visible layer of cells in the anterior chamber, is a characteristic sign of ocular Behcet's disease. Other ocular lesions include iridocyclitis, scleritis, keratitis, vitreous hemorrhage, optic neuritis, retinal vein occlusion, and retinal neovascularization.

Skin disease occurs in about 80% of patients with Behcet's disease, and lesions often occur in combination. Erythema nodosum is common, particularly in females. It usually affects the lower limbs and may resolve leaving hyperpigmented areas. Superficial thrombophlebitis is also common and may be confused with erythema nodosum. Papulopustular lesions and acneiform nodules also occur.

Pathergy is the name given to nonspecific hyperreactivity of the skin following minor trauma, which is specific to Behcet's disease.

Joint manifestations are very common in Behcet's disease, occurring in almost two-thirds of patients. The most frequent manifestation is a nonerosive, nondeforming oligoarthralgia, typically involving the knees, ankles, and wrists.

Venous involvement is more common and may result in both superficial thrombophlebitis and deep venous thrombosis.

Involvement of the CNS occurs in 5–10% of patients. Neurological manifestations usually occurs within 5 years of disease onset and are most common in men.

Parenchymal brain involvement is most common (80%) and particularly affects the brainstem. Nonparenchymal disease, including dural sinus thrombosis, aseptic meningitis, and arterial vasculitis, may also occur.

The involvement of the gastrointestinal tract is variable. The spectrum of clinical symptom is wide and includes anorexia, vomiting, dyspepsia, diarrhea, and abdominal pain. Indeed, Behcet's disease shares many of the features of the inflammatory bowel diseases.

Differential Diagnosis

The differential diagnosis includes: Reiter's syndrome may be associated with oral and genital ulcers, although the arthritis is generally erosive. Urethritis and sacroiliitis are not features of Behcet's disease. Stevens-Johnson syndrome also presents with mucocutaneous involvement and conjunctivitis, but is not associated with thrombophlebitis, uveitis or, arterial disease.

Recurrent orogenital ulceration may also be associated with bullous skin disorders and erythema multiforme.

Pyoderma gangrenosum (PG) can present with genital ulcers. Classic pyoderma gangrenosum is characterized by a deep ulceration with a violaceous border that overhangs the ulcer bed. These lesions of PG most commonly occur on the legs, but they may occur anywhere on the body (Figs 18 and 19). PG may occur

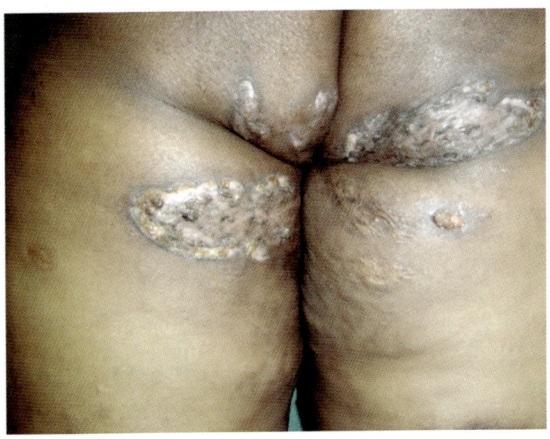

Figure 18: Pyoderma gangrenosum in female who had extensive lesions

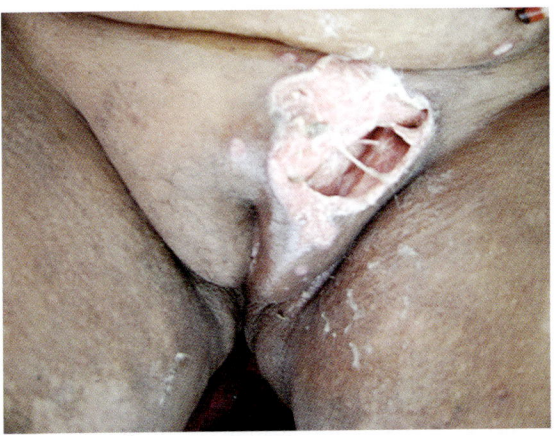

Figure 19: Pyoderma gangrenosum of the genitals in a child

on the genitalia. This form, termed vulvar or penile PG, must be differentiated from sexually transmitted diseases.

Treatment

The primary goals of management are symptom control, early suppression of inflammation, and prevention of end-organ damage, the treatment options being anti-inflammatory agents and immunosuppressants.

Oral ulceration can often be treated by the topical application of corticosteroids, using creams or mouthwashes. Similarly, genital ulceration often responds to topical corticosteroid therapy, although long-term use may be complicated by skin atrophy.

Systemic corticosteroids are frequently used in the management of acute disease exacerbations. Other systemic therapies include: cyclosporine, methotrexate, cyclophosphamide, azathioprine, dapsone, thalidomide, pentoxifylline, infliximab, etanercept, and interferon-α.

BALANOPOSTHITIS

Balanitis is defined as inflammation of the glans penis, which often involves the prepuce (Fig. 20). There is a wide variety of causes and predisposing factors; it is more common among uncircumcised men possibly as a result of poorer hygiene and aeration or because of irritation by smegma. Underlying medical conditions can also predispose to balanitis, which may be more severe. Inflammation of the glans and prepuce may also provide a route for the acquisition of the human immunodeficiency virus (HIV) infection.

Causative factors of balanoposthitis are given in Table 1.

Fungal

Candidal balanitis is considered to be the most common cause of balanitis and is due to infection with candidal species, usually *Candida albicans*. It is generally sexually acquired, although carriage of yeasts on the penis is common, being 14–18% with no significant differences between carriage rate in circumcised and uncircumcised

Inflammatory Lesions of the Genitalia

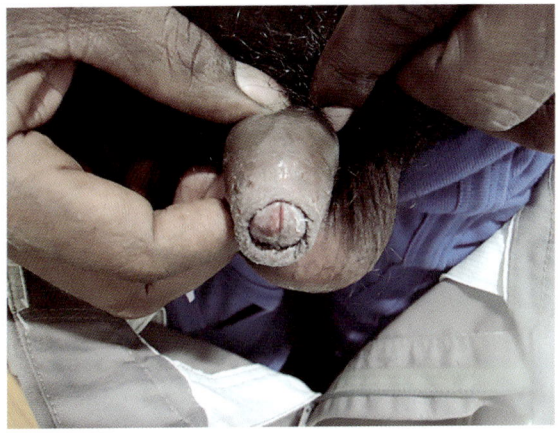

Figure 20: Balanoposthitis showing inflammation of glans and prepuce

TABLE 1: Causative factors of balanoposthitis

Infectionsl	Dermatoses	Miscellaneous
Candida albicans	Lichen sclerosus (balanitis xerotica obliterans)	Trauma
Trichomonas vaginalis	Zoon's balanitis	Irritant
Streptococci (Group A and B)	Psoriasis	Poor hygiene
Anaerobes	Circinate balanitis	Premalignant conditions: Bowen's disease Bowenoid papulosis Erythroplasia of Queyrat
Gardnerella vaginalis	Lichen planus	
Staphylococcus aureus	Immunobullous disorders	
Mycobacteria	Contact allergy	
Entamoeba histolytica	Fixed drug eruption	
Syphilis	Stevens Johnson Syndrome	
Herpes simplex virus, human papilloma virus		

men. Symptomatic infection is more common in the uncircumcised male. Significantly, more of the female partners of men carrying yeasts were found to have candidal infection. Diagnosis may be on clinical appearances alone, microscopy, and/or culture. The sensitivity of microscopy varies with method of sampling, and an "adhesive tape" method has proven to be more accurate than swabbing. Infection may occur without sexual contact, usually in the presence of diabetes of which it may be the presenting symptom, or after the use of oral antibiotics. Symptoms are burning and itching of the penis with generalized erythema of the glans and/or prepuce which may have a dry glazed appearance, with eroded white papules and white discharge. In diabetic patients, the presentation may be more severe with edema and fissuring of the foreskin, which may become nonretractile. Treatment can be topical (for example clotrimazole), or oral (such as fluconazole), but partners should be screened as they may have a high rate of infection.

Anaerobic Infection

The presence of anaerobes on the glans penis, particularly in the uncircumcised male has been associated with nonspecific urethritis (NSU) and balanitis. A severe erosive and gangrenous form of anaerobic balanitis (the fourth venereal disease of Corbus) has been recognized for many years with the presence of anaerobes and *Fusobacterium* spp. Anaerobes do not appear to cause genital ulceration, but are found in genital ulcers of any etiology, and in this situation the predominant strains are: *Bacteroides ureolyticus* and *asaccharolytica*. The features of anaerobic balanitis are superficial erosions, foul-smelling subpreputial discharge, preputial edema, and inguinal adenitis. More minor forms also occur. Resolution is normally rapid with metronidazole treatment.

Aerobic Infection

Gardnerella vaginalis is likely to be sexually acquired and partners of women with *G. vaginalis* have high isolation rates from the urethra or urine. Subpreputial carriage in consorts of women with *G. vaginalis* have not been studied specifically.

The symptoms of pure *G. vaginalis* balanitis are milder than those in anaerobic infection with irritation of the prepuce and glans penis, macular erythema and, a fishy subpreputial discharge. As co-infection with anaerobes is common, this may represent the milder end of a spectrum of disease.

Streptococci, group B *streptococci* can be carried asymptomatically in the adult genital tract, but are strongly associated with balanitis. Sexual transmission is unclear as there was no expected age differential in one study, and in another meatal carriage was not proportional to promiscuity. The clinical appearance is of nonspecific erythema. Penicillins or cephalosporins are effective in treatment.

Staphyloccocus aureus has infrequently been reported as causing balanitis, although carriage is not strongly associated with symptoms.

Mycobacterial

Tuberculosis presents as a chronic popular eruption of the glans penis, which may be ulcerated, and heals with scarring. It is associated with a positive Mantoux test and histology shows tuberculoid granuloma formation with a characteristic absence of tubercle bacilli. Penis tuberculides are thought to be due to the hematogenous spread of infection, and respond well to antituberculous chemotherapy.

Leprosy involvement of the glans penis has been reported in leprosy alone and in association with penis tuberculides.

Protozoal

Trichomonas: Trichomonas can cause a sexually acquired superficial erosive balanitis which may lead to phimosis. There is a strong association with the presence of other infections. Histology of the lesions shows dense lymphocytic infiltration in the upper dermis. The organism may be demonstrated in a wet preparation from the subpreputial sac. This condition responds well to treatment with metronidazole.

Entamoeba histolytica: Cutaneous amoebiasis of the genitalia occurs occasionally, and amoebic balanitis has been reported among uncircumcised men in New Guinea. It causes edema of the prepuce with phimosis and discharge, and in those cases circumcision is helpful.

Spirochetal

Syphilitic balanitis: Multiple circinate lesions which erode to cause irregular ulcers have been described in the late primary or early secondary stage. A primary chancre may also be present. Spirochetes are easily identified from the lesions.

Nonsyphilitic spirochetes: Ulcerative balanitis has been associated with infection by nonsyphilitic treponemes of the borrelia group, and spirochetes have been observed on dark-field microscopy. This often co-exists with other genital infection, and has been reported from Africa and India.

Viral Infection

Herpes simplex: In rare cases, primary herpes can cause a necrotizing balanitis, with necrotic areas on the glans accompanied by vesicles elsewhere, and associated with headache and malaise. This has been reported with HSV types 1 and 2.

Human papillomavirus (HPV): Papillomavirus may be associated with a patchy or chronic balanitis, which becomes acetowhite after the application of 5% acetic acid. Acetowhite change has also been reported in non-HPV associated balanitis and has resolved on treatment.

Irritant and Allergic Balanitis

Many balanitis are nonspecific and no etiological agent can be found. It has been suggested that these are often due to irritation, particularly, if symptoms are persistent or recurrent. In one study of patients with persistent or recurrent problems 72% were diagnosed with irritant balanitis, and this was associated with a history of atopy and more frequent genital washing with soap. Other series have found higher rates of infective agents, although a large proportion of cases in one study remained undiagnosed. It is likely that irritation plays some part in other balanitis. More severe reactions have been seen with topical agents, some of which may have been used for treatment. Dequalinium is known to cause a necrotic balanitis, while titanium (that was previously thought to be biologically inert) may cause a necrotic balanitis. Balanitis as an allergic reaction is very uncommon; rubber and its constituents are the most frequently described allergens, although allergy to spermicidal lubricants is also well described. There is a wide spectrum of clinical manifestations varying from balanitis to edema of the whole penis extending to the groins. Treatment will depend on the severity of the reaction, but patch testing and avoidance of the precipitant is required.

PLASMA CELL BALANITIS (ZOON'S BALANITIS)

A disorder first described by Zoon in 1952, Zoon's balanitis (ZB) or plasma cell balanitis (PCB), is a chronic, benign, rare inflammatory disorder that manifests as lesions localized on the glans penis and prepuce, seen in middle-aged uncircumcised men.

Etiology

The etiology of the condition is not clearly established. It has been mostly found in uncircumcised men; besides heat, friction, hypospadia, and lack of genital hygiene are believed to be predisposing factors. Trauma may be a contributory cause, as localization of the lesions is mostly on the dorsal site of the glans and prepuce, which is more commonly subjected to minor trauma than the ventral site. Retention of smegma and formation of "smegma stones" have been repeatedly described in patients with phimosis in whom retention of urine may lead to constant irritation of the skin.

Some authors suggest that balanitis represents a nonspecific inflammatory response to an unknown exogenous agent, and therefore is associated with plasma cell infiltration predominated by IgG producing cells, suggesting a nonspecific polyclonal stimulation of B-cells, as is common in chronic infections. Chronic infection by *Mycobacterium smegmatis* and HPV has been postulated; however, no evidence has yet been reported.

Genital Dermatoses

Clinical Features

There are well-defined, red, shiny plaques on the glans penis or inner surface of the foreskin. (Fig. 21). Patients may have single or multiple lesions, and often a lesion on the glans is mirrored on the inner surface of the adjacent prepuce.

Cayenne pepper spots occur within the plaque, which represent dilated capillaries, and may be associated with a brownish color from hemosiderin deposition.

There are often no symptoms, or the patient notices a slight sticky discharge from the involved mucosa. There may be slight irritation, but a feature is that it is relatively asymptomatic for such a dramatic appearance.

Pathology

Diagnosis is confirmed by the distinctive histologic findings. Epidermal atrophy with complete effacement of the rete ridges is present. Ulceration may occur. Suprabasal keratinocytes are diamond-shaped, which are also called "lozenge keratinocytes", are common with uniform intercellular spaces termed "watery spongiosis." A dense, lichenoid, subepidermal infiltrate composed

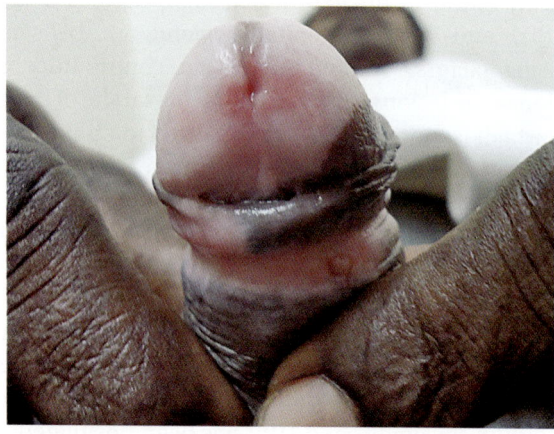

Figure 21: Well defined, red, shiny plaques on the glans penis and inner surface of the foreskin of Zoon's balanitis

largely of plasma cells is characteristic. Erythrocyte extravasation and hemosiderin deposition are often noted.

Differential Diagnosis

Zoon's balanitis can at times be difficult to distinguish from other erythematous lesions involving the balanopreputial sac [e.g. erythroplasia of Queyrat (EQ), localized forms of LP, cicatricial pemphigoid, unilesional forms of psoriasis, syphilis, candidiasis], and therefore can be easily misdiagnosed. Other conditions in the differential diagnosis are contact dermatitis, SCC, LSA, and balanitis xerotica obliterans. Biopsy is necessary to help clarify the nature of the disease. Microscopy for fungi, Tzanck smear, viral, bacterial and fungal cultures, fasting blood glucose measurement, and serology for syphilis are other tests that may be used to help rule out other causes.

Treatment

The initial treatment regimen may include good hygiene, emollient creams, and topical corticosteroids. Circumcision is usually curative. Tacrolimus is an alternative treatment for patients in whom there is good reason to avoid topical corticosteroids and for those who refuse surgery. Other options include topical fusidic acid and imiquimod. Successful ablation of PCB has been achieved with carbon dioxide laser and erbium: yttrium aluminium garnet (YAG) laser.

Reiter's Syndrome

Reiter's syndrome is a multisystem disease, characterized classically as a triad of nongonococcal urethritis, conjunctivitis, and arthritis in association with the mucocutaneous lesions of keratoderma blennorrhagica, and balanitis circinata. The fact only one-third of patients show the complete triad and the recognition of incomplete Reiter's syndrome prompted the American Rheumatism Association to define Reiter's syndrome as "an episode of peripheral arthritis of more than one month's duration occurring in association with urethritis and/or cervicitis".

Etiology

The exact cause of Reiter's syndrome is unknown. It often begins following a bacterial infection in the intestine (*Salmonella, Shigella, Campylobacter* or *Yersinia*) or genitourinary tract (*Chlamydia*). It is not known exactly why some people exposed to certain bacteria develop the disorder and others do not. However, the presence of a certain gene HLA-B27 increases a person's likelihood of developing Reiter's syndrome.

Pathogenesis and Clinical Features

Reiter's syndrome is a multisystem disease commonly triggered by a genitourinary infection, such as chlamydia, or a bacterial enteric infection caused by *Shigella, Campylobacter*, or *Salmonella*. It has been postulated that bacterial antigens persist within the synovium and other tissues, stimulating a proliferative T-cell response. This proliferative T-cell response eventually targets autoantigens, causing inflammation and tissue destruction. After a latent period of 1 week to 1 month, ocular symptoms develop, such as sterile conjunctivitis or iritis, combined with oligoarthritis. The oligoarthritis is usually asymmetric and affects the lower extremities, including the knees or ankles. Enthesopathy or inflammation of tendons at their insertions, especially the Achilles tendon and dactylitis, or "sausage digits", may also occur. Constitutional symptoms, such as fever and weight loss, are not uncommon during the acute phase of Reiter's syndrome.

Mucocutaneous involvement occurs in approximately 50% of patients with Reiter's syndrome. It may occur before or after the onset of oligoarthritis. The two classic cutaneous manifestations of Reiter's syndrome are keratoderma blennorrhagicum and balanitis circinata, both of which are microscopically similar to pustular psoriasis. Keratoderma blennorrhagicum appears 1–2 months after the onset of arthritis and is present in about 10% of patients. It almost always involves the soles, but may affect the legs, hands, nails, and scalp. Keratoderma blennorrhagicum typically begins as a red macule or vesicle and evolves into a hyperkeratotic papule or plaque.

The mature lesion appears as a crusted, hyperkeratotic plaque that grossly resembles psoriasis. Nail involvement is also common and may begin as painless, red swelling along the nail fold followed by a thickening of the nail plate. Subungual pustules and onycholysis also may occur.

Balanitis circinata occurs in about 25% of men with Reiter's syndrome. In uncircumcised men, shallow, erythematous, eroded plaques or ulcers may form on the glans penis. These lesions typically have well-defined borders and are often in a circinate configuration. In circumcised men, the erosions may develop into thick hyperkeratotic plaques and also may involve the penile shaft or scrotum. Similar lesions also may affect the vulva or vaginal mucosa in women.

Oral involvement occurs in 15–30% of affected patients, appearing as transient, asymptomatic vesicles or ulcers on the soft palate, uvula, tongue, or buccal mucosa.

Laboratory Findings

Laboratory findings in patients with Reiter's syndrome are generally nonspecific and may include mild anemia, elevated erythrocyte sedimentation rate, and increased C-reactive protein. Synovial fluid analysis of the arthritic joints demonstrates a sterile, inflammatory synovitis with 15,000–30,000 neutrophils/μL. Reiter's syndrome has been linked with HLA-B27 positivity, but evidence suggests this association may be related to more severe and chronic forms of the disease.

Treatment

Treatment for the joint symptoms of Reiter's syndrome includes NSAIDs, such as indomethacin, and intra-articular steroids. The skin manifestations may be treated in a similar fashion to psoriasis, using topical steroids, ultraviolet B (UVB) phototherapy, coal tar, and etretinate. In persistent or severe disease, immunosuppressive agents such as azathioprine, sulfasalazine, methotrexate, or oral corticosteroids may be used.

Genital Dermatoses

PSORIASIS

Psoriasis is an inflammatory skin disease that typically follows a relapsing and remitting course.

Clinical Features

Psoriatic lesions on the genital skin often present as well-demarcated, brightly erythematous, thin plaques, and usually lack, due to maceration, the typical scaling that is apparent on other parts of the body. However, scales may be seen on the more keratinized regions of the genital skin. When scaling is present, it is often minimal and can easily be scraped off, leaving pinpoint bleedings. The appearance of vulvar psoriasis is often symmetrical and can vary from silvery, scaling patches adjacent to the outer parts of the labia majora to moist grayish plaques or glossy red plaques without scaling in the skin folds. In male patients, both scrotal and penile skin may be affected (Figs 22 to 32). The glans penis is the area of male genital skin that is most commonly affected. Occasionally, the entire penis, scrotum, and inguinal folds are involved. Whereas in uncircumcised males, the well-defined, nonscaling plaques are most common under the prepuce and on the proximal glans; in

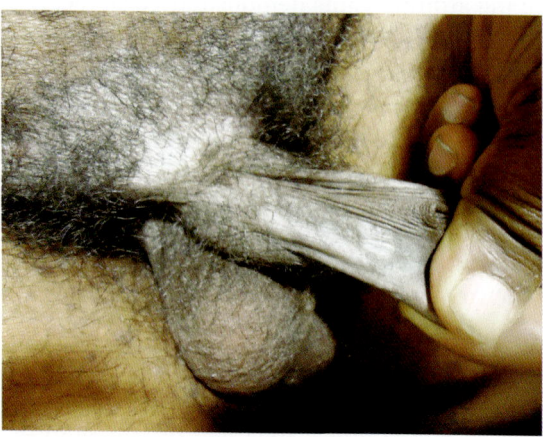

Figure 22: Dry scaly plaque of psoriasis

Inflammatory Lesions of the Genitalia

circumcised male patients, the lesions are usually present on the glans and corona. Psoriatic genital lesions of the glans and corona in circumcised males can be more scalier than those usually seen

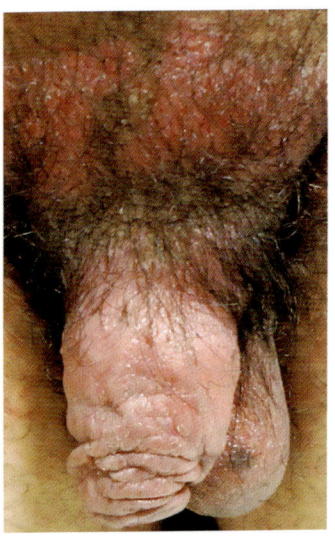

Figure 23: Classical erythematous plaques involving the penile and scrotal skin

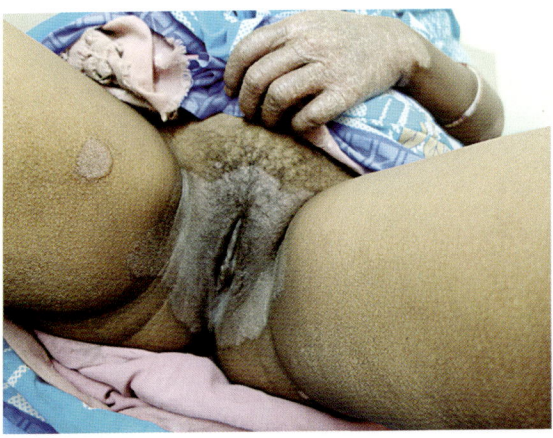

Figure 24: Flexural psoriasis in a woman

Genital Dermatoses

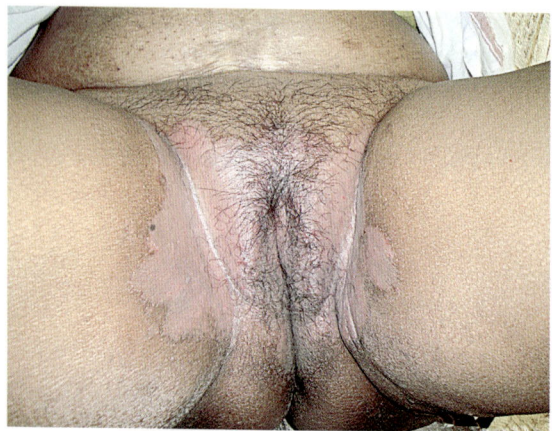

Figure 25: Flexural psoriasis in an old lady involving the groin and the labial skin

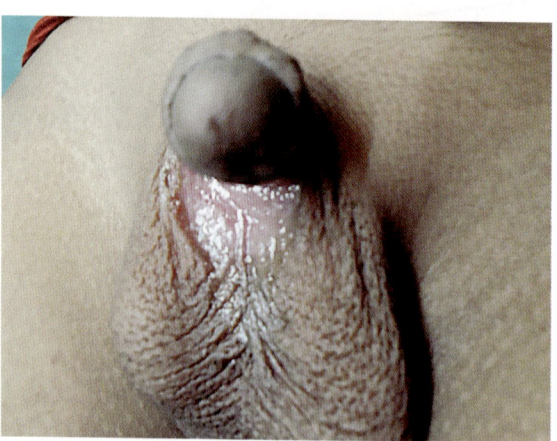

Figure 26: Genital psoriasis with super added candidal infection

in genital skin. Patients with genital psoriasis may also experience pruritus and/or a burning sensation in the affected area, which can range from minimal to marked. Due to the Koebner phenomenon, genital psoriasis may be worsened by irritation from urine and feces, tight-fitting clothes, and sexual intercourse.

Inflammatory Lesions of the Genitalia

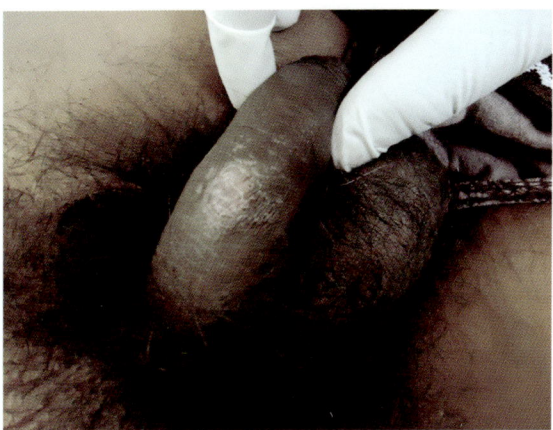

Figure 27: Isolated genital involvement easy to miss. Patient later developed extensive psoriasis vulgaris

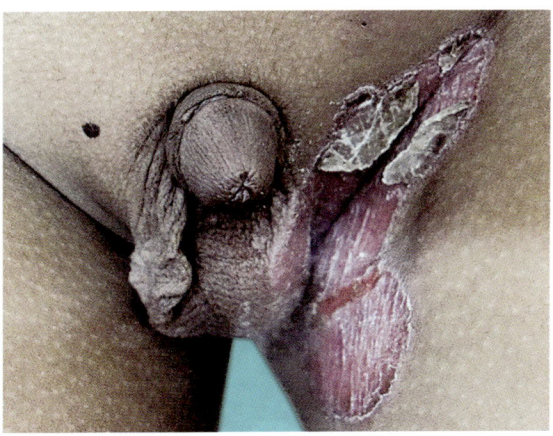

Figure 28: Psoriasis involving the groin in a child

Diagnosis

Genital psoriatic lesions may be the only psoriatic feature in a particular patient, but more often they are part of a more generalized form of psoriasis. Confirmatory lesions elsewhere or other clinical signs of psoriasis (such as nail deformities or joint complaints) may be present.

Genital Dermatoses

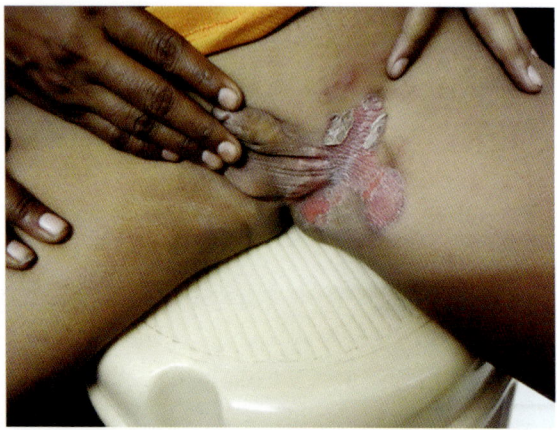

Figure 29: Psoriasis involving the groin, note the fissure

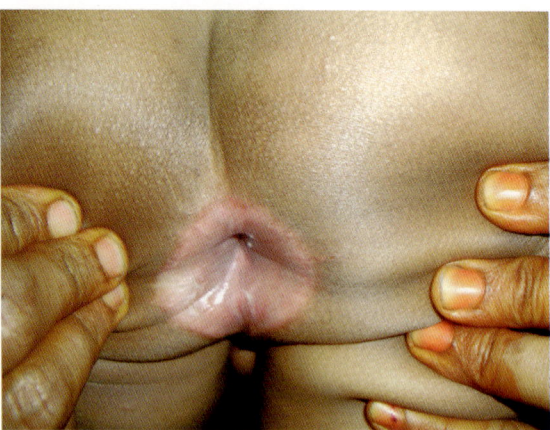

Figure 30: Involvement of perianal area in an infant with genital psoriasis

Histologically, there is no apparent difference between genital and nongenital psoriasis. However, the typical characteristics of psoriasis may be less evident in vulvar and penile psoriatic lesions, which may necessitate a careful search for subtle signs in these cases.

Inflammatory Lesions of the Genitalia

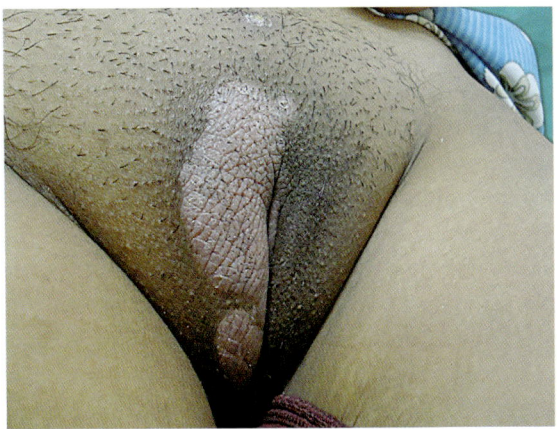

Figure 31: Psoriatic plaque with pink hue and lichenification secondary to scratching

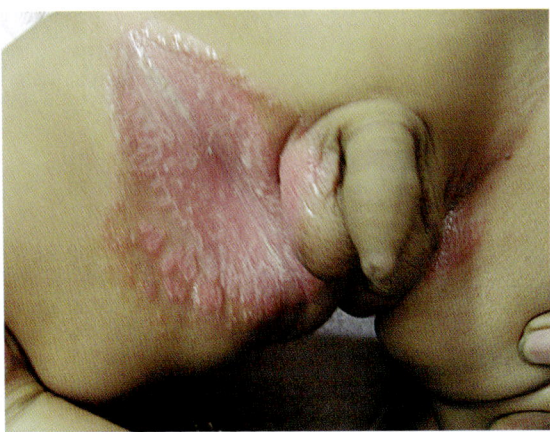

Figure 32: Psoriasis involving the groin, thigh, and the scrotal skin

Treatment

Most of the authors are reluctant in the prescription of corticosteroids for genital psoriasis and only recommend the use of mild (and sometimes, if necessary, moderate) steroids.

Vitamin D analogues are another possible nonsteroidal treatment for genital psoriatic lesions, in particular those affecting male genital skin. They can be prescribed as monotherapy or in combination with steroid preparations. Vitamin D analogues may cause irritation, which may be minimized by their combination with steroids.

Pimecrolimus ointment or tacrolimus cream may be useful, while acknowledging that they may cause local irritation and stinging.

Suspected concurrent bacterial or fungal infections of the genital area should be treated with topical antibiotics or ketoconazole or miconazole, respectively, to eliminate the possible Koebner effect.

Moreover, minimizing contact with local irritating factors and the use of mild emollients may be useful in the treatment of genital psoriasis.

Systemic therapy is no common practice for isolated genital psoriasis. Nevertheless, such treatment modalities may also be beneficial for genital lesions, if prescribed, because of severe and extensive psoriasis.

Anthralin, tazarotene, UV-light, and laser therapy should be avoided in the genital area.

ECZEMA

Eczema on the genitals may be classified as exogenous (allergic contact dermatitis or irritant contact dermatitis) or endogenous (atopic eczema or seborrheic eczema). Other forms of eczema on the genitals are exceptionally rare. Diaper dermatitis is a distint entity involving the diaper area (Figs 33 to 44).

Allergic Contact Dermatitis

As the name suggests, this form of eczema is caused by direct contact with a sensitizing substance. The reaction is in the form of a type IV (delayed type) hypersensitivity. Allergens may be applied directly to the skin (for example in the form of a cream), or may be transferred from elsewhere (for example by the hands after handling an allergic substance).

Inflammatory Lesions of the Genitalia

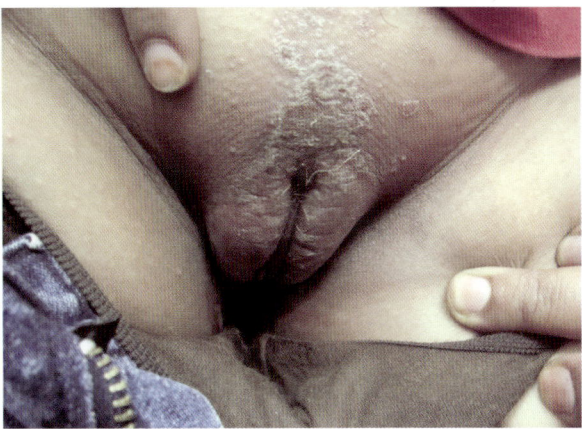

Figure 33: Contact eczema leading to lichenification

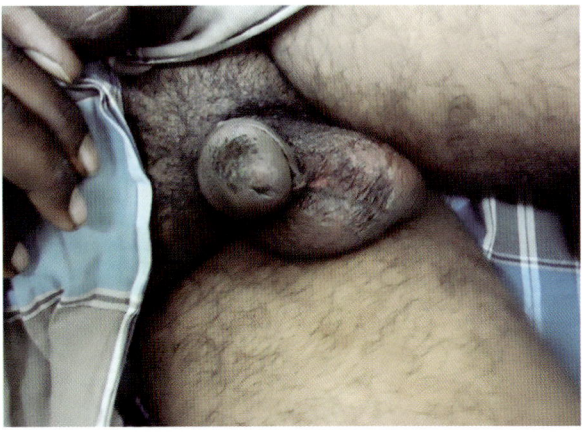

Figure 34: Contact dermatitis of scrotal skin due to Dettol, note erythema and erosions over scrotum and shaft of penis

Symptoms may be acute, chronic, or acute-on-chronic. Acute contact dermatitis of the genital skin usually presents with redness, itching, and swelling. In severe cases, the skin may blister and there may be exudation. This reaction tends to occur within 24-48 hours after contact with a sensitizing agent. With intermittent exposure to

Genital Dermatoses

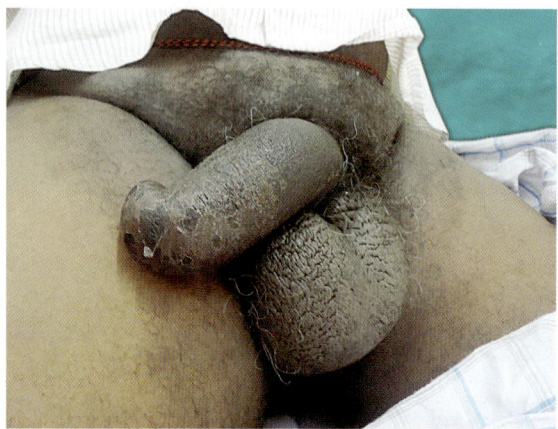

Figure 35: Irritant contact dermatitis involving the scrotal and penile skin

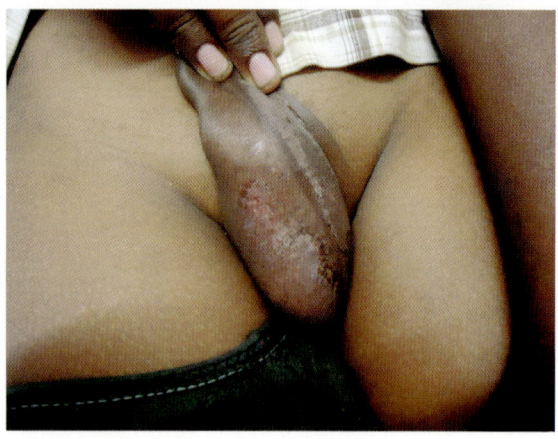

Figure 36: Scrotal eczema in an atopic child

an offending allergen, a chronic, irritating, and lichenified eczema may develop.

Investigation with patch testing is essential. Treatment involves withdrawing offending allergens, if known, avoiding irritants (such

Inflammatory Lesions of the Genitalia

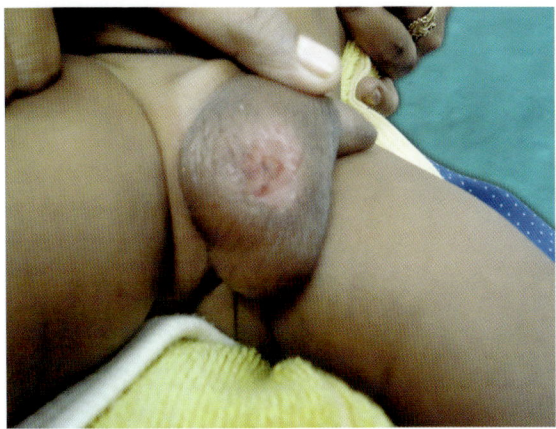

Figure 37: Eczematous rash in an atopic child due to constant wearing of diaper

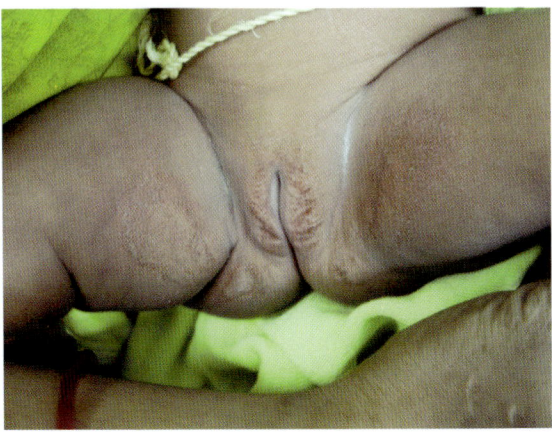

Figure 38: Diaper dermatitis involving the convexities where there is direct contact with diaper. Note the sparing of folds

as soap) and the use of moderately potent topical steroids for limited periods.

Type IV reactions to latex may occur, but are relatively rare. Type I reactions to rubber in the form of latex reactions are important since

Genital Dermatoses

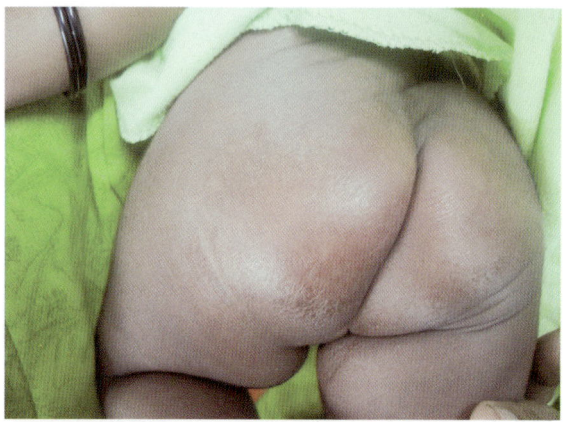

Figure 39: Erythema typical of diaper dermatitis

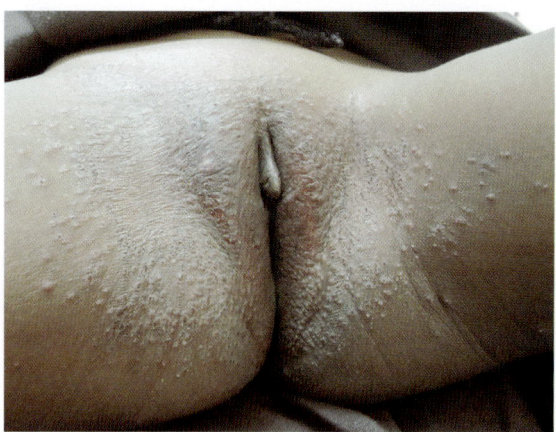

Figure 40: Erythematous papules and scaling of irritant dermatitis due to savlon

they may be very severe or even life-threatening. These reactions may cause acute (within minutes) urticaria, swelling, irritation, and redness of the skin, but may also precipitate acute anaphylaxis.

Inflammatory Lesions of the Genitalia

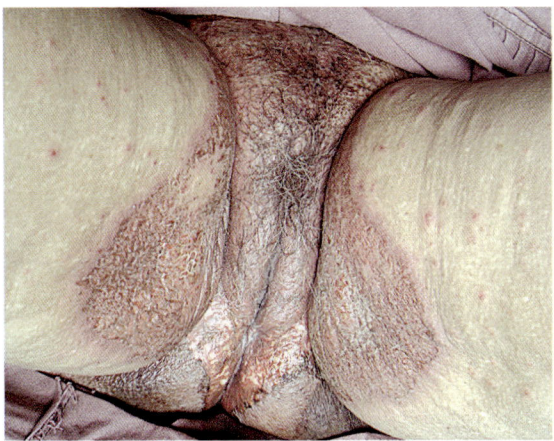

Figure 41: Irritant contact dermatits in an elderly woman involving the entire perineal skin and part of thigh

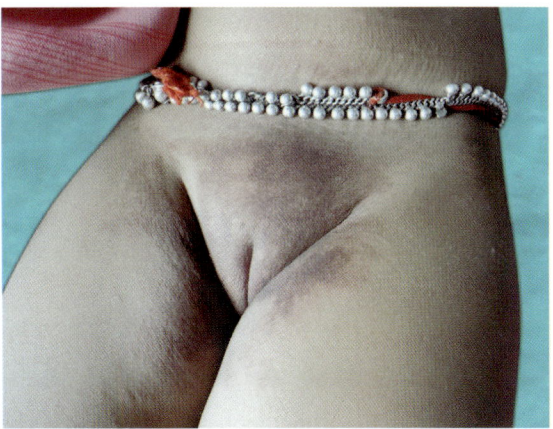

Figure 42: Irritant dermatitis of diaper area in a child showing involvement of the convexities

Irritant Contact Dermatitis

Irritant contact dermatitis may be clinically indistinguishable from allergic contact dermatitis. There are a large number of potential

Genital Dermatoses

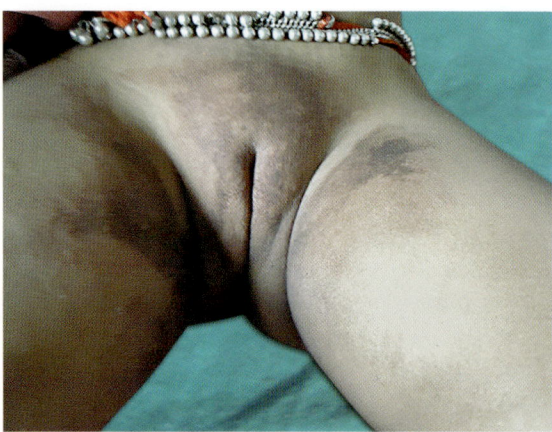

Figure 43: Same as in 42 showing sparing concavities

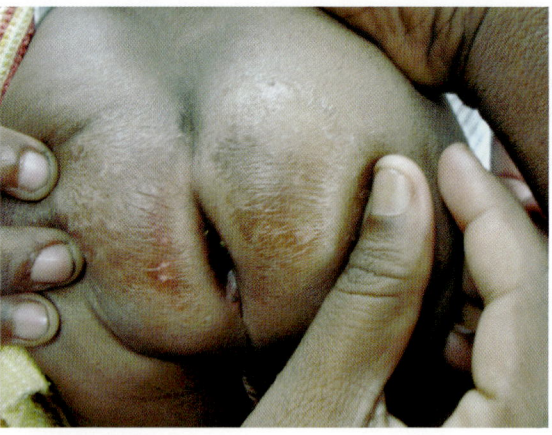

Figure 44: Note the sparing of the perianal area diaper contact dermatitis

irritants (see below), particularly soaps, shower gels, and bath products which are often highly fragranced. Poor hygiene is often a predisposing factor, especially in older men.

Typical irritants of the genital area:
- Soaps, shower gels, and other toiletries

Inflammatory Lesions of the Genitalia

TABLE 2: Common sources of allergic contact dermatitis on the genitalia

Where allergen originates from	Source	Examples	Specific sensitizers
Direct contact	Medicaments and skin-care products	Topical steroids, emollients, local anesthetic creams, antibiotics, antifungals, bath products	Parabens, ethylenediamine, sorbic acid, propylene glycol, etc.
	Contraceptives	Condoms	Latex, spermicides, rubber chemicals
Allergen transfer	Hands Partner	Industrial allergens Feminine products	Nickel, epoxies Fragrances

- Urine, and feces
- Sweat, and sebum
- Condoms, spermicides, and products to enhance sex
- Sexual secretions
- Tight clothing and friction.
- Externally applied medication for diseases of the genital skin

Management of irritant contact dermatitis is similar to that of allergic contact dermatitis with avoidance of all irritant factors, use of appropriate emollients and soap substitutes, and limited use of a topical steroid. Sometimes, folliculitis due to secondary bacterial infection can be a complication of irritant contact dermatitis which will require antibiotics either topical or systemic.

Common sources of allergic contact dermatitis on the genitalia are given in Table 2.

Atopic Eczema and Lichen Simplex

Atopic eczema (atopic dermatitis) is very common, affecting around 10% of children, although only a small percentage will continue to have problems into adulthood. In moderate and severe cases, the

Genital Dermatoses

eruption may be widespread and affect the genital area. It is unusual for atopic eczema to be only confined to the genitals and lesions will invariably be visible elsewhere on the body. These groups of patients are more prone to contact allergy (see above) and patch testing may be useful in their management. Treatment is the same for allergic contact dermatitis and irritant contact dermatitis.

Lichen simplex is the term given to describe chronic, lichenified eczema of any variety. It is very common in the groins and on the scrotum where it is produced by scratching and rubbing. It may develop into intertrigo and may be complicated by bacterial or fungal infection, particularly in the groins. General advice, such as keeping the fingernails short is important. Treatment is similar to that of the other forms of eczema but due to the intense itch, potent topical steroids may be necessary for a longer period. Secondary infection should be treated concurrently.

Seborrheic Eczema (Seborrheic Dermatitis)

Seborrheic eczema is a papulosquamous skin disorder, usually localized to specific sebum-rich areas of the body such as the face, scalp, and trunk, but also occurs in hairy areas such as the pubic area. It occurs worldwide and at a higher rate in men than women. The prevalence is estimated at around 5% in healthy individuals but occurs in up to 85% of HIV-infected patients. It is associated with an abnormal immune response to the *Malassezia* yeast species.

Symptoms may be mild or absent. Mild itching, tingling, or even burning of the skin may occur. Erythema, scaling, and crusting are present to variable degrees. The eruption may be confined to the genital area, but closer examination will often reveal signs elsewhere, such as dandruff in the scalp and mild scaling affecting the nasolabial folds, eyebrows, and eyelash areas.

Seborrheic eczema is usually the first cutaneous manifestation of HIV infection. In long-standing HIV infection where immune function is severely compromised, seborrheic eczema may be very severe or generalized.

Diagnosis is usually made clinically, but skin scrapings may be necessary to exclude tinea. The yeast will be visible on microscopy. The differential diagnosis includes genital psoriasis (which may also co-exist), other forms of eczema, and fungal infections. Standard therapies tend to combine a mild topical steroid with an antifungal agent, as well as the use of emollients and soap substitutes. Unfortunately, the yeast cannot be completely eradicated and the eruption tends to recur periodically.

Diaper Dermatitis (Diaper rash)

The term, diaper rash, or diaper dermatitis, encompasses all inflammatory skin conditions that can occur in the diaper area. The distinguishing clinical finding is the sparing of folds where the diaper does not come into contact with. These disorders occurring in the diaper area can be conceptually divided into following categories:
- Rashes that are caused by the wearing of diapers, namely irritant contact dermatitis, miliaria, intertrigo, candidal diaper dermatitis, and granuloma gluteal infantum
- Rashes that are exaggerated due to the irritating effects of wearing a diaper that includes atopic dermatitis, seborrheic dermatitis, and psoriasis
- Rashes that appear irrespective of diaper use, which will mean rashes due to bullous impetigo, Letterer-Siwe disease, acrodermatitis enteropathica, and congenital syphilis.

Treatment

Changes in diapering practices and keeping the skin in the diaper area dry are the mainstay of management. Liquid paraffin, petrolatum ointment, cream containing zinc oxide will offer more protection. Antifungal and antibacterial agents are required whenever there is super-added fungal or bacterial infection. Irritant dermatitis can be treated with nonfluorinated, low-potency corticosteroid cream for no longer than 2 weeks.

SQUAMOUS CELL HYPERPLASIA

Squamous cell hyperplasia (with and without atypia) (Figs 45 to 49) is not a distinct entity, it is only a description of a morphologic alteration of vulvar skin. It is commonly seen in premenopausal

Genital Dermatoses

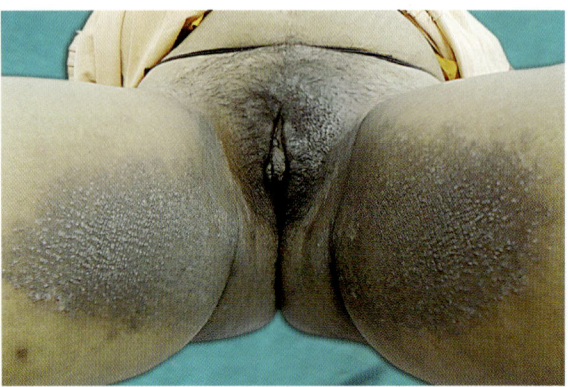

Figure 45: Squamous hyperplasia mimicking lichen simplex

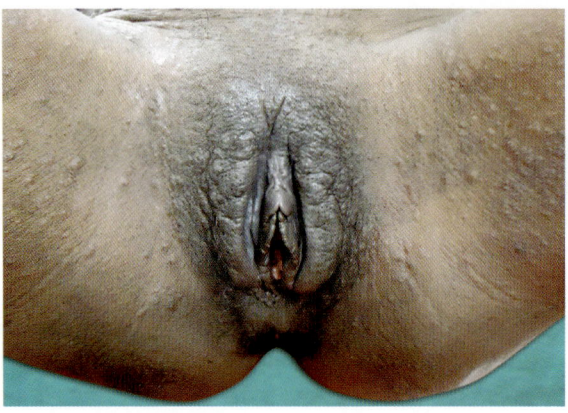

Figure 46: Squamous cell hyperplasia in a pregnant woman

women. It presents with pruritus followed by a cycle of itching, scrubbing, and scratching leading to lichenification. Sometimes, secondary changes due to superadded infection, resulting from trauma, caused by scratching, may be evident. It is a diagnosis of exclusion on the basis of specific anatomical and clinical features. This entity has been observed frequently in pregnant women. Squamous cell hyperplasaia is related to chronic irritation and is not

Inflammatory Lesions of the Genitalia

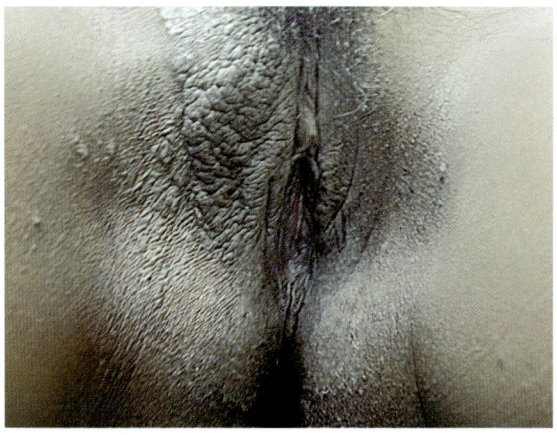

Figure 47: Squamous cell hyperplasia occurring in a background of lichen sclerosus

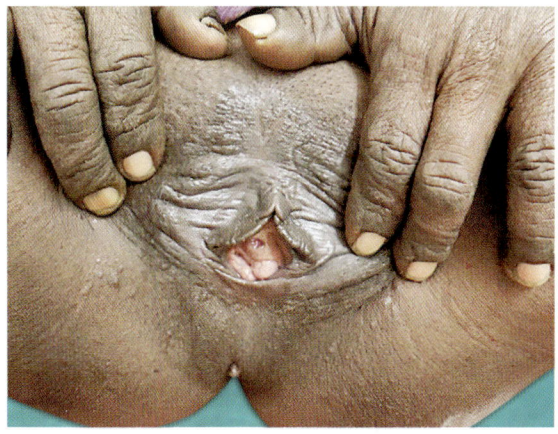

Figure 48: Squamous hyperplasia in a multiparous woman

a precursor to HIV negative SCC. Histologically, it is characterized by hyperkeratosis, which is a prominent feature, sometimes, parakeratosis may be present. Elongation and widening of the rete ridges with irregular acanthosis and chronic inflammation in dermis

Genital Dermatoses

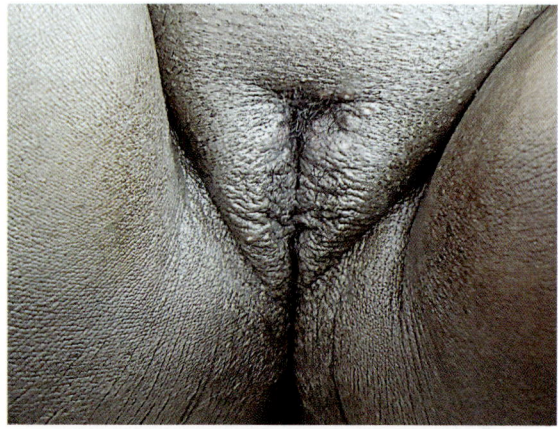

Figure 49: Squamous hyperplasia with secondary changes

are regular observations. Sometimes, may have increased mitotic figures in basal and prickle cell, but atypia is not a feature. However, squamous cell hyperplasia, occurring in a background of lichen sclerosus, constitutes a distinct group at higher risk of developing invasive cancer. Judicious use of topical corticosteroids will relieve itching. In pregnant women, this condition reverts to normal, few months after delivery.

VITILIGO

Vitiligo can affect any body parts, including the genital skin and mucosa as a depigmented macule or patch. Skin of scrotum, penis, glans in males and vulva, vagina, and labia in females are the sites of involvement (Figs 50 to 53). The genitals affected with vitiligo falls in the 'mucocutaneous' category, where skin and mucus membrane meet. This variety of vitiligo is difficult to cure. One has to work on controlling spread. Vitiligo can occur together with lichen sclerosus.

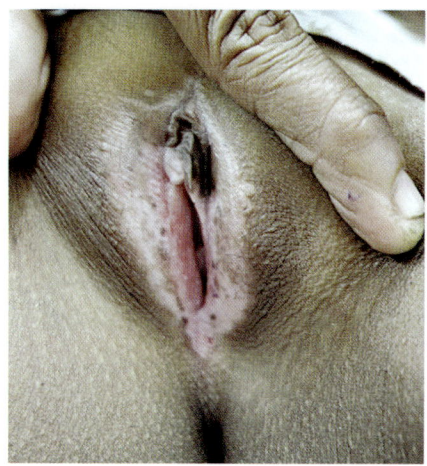

Figure 50: Vitiligo showing spots of repigmentation

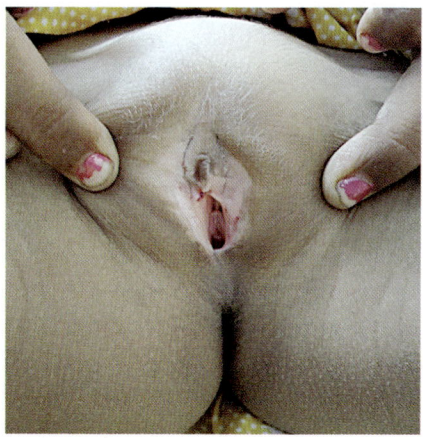

Figure 51: Vitiligo with leucotrichia indicating gaurded prognosis

Close monitoring of patients with genital vitiligo is important in order to make early diagnosis of LSA, which is a premalignant condition in some.

Genital Dermatoses

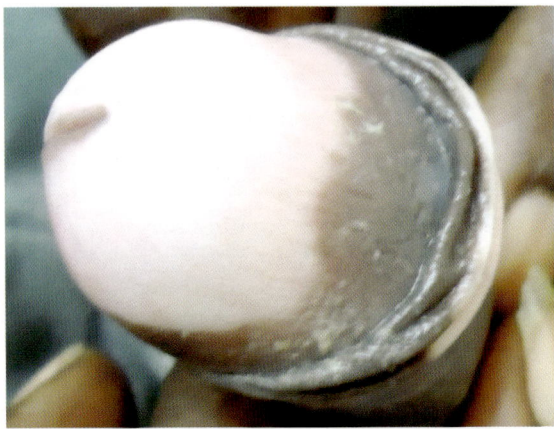

Figure 52: Vitiligo of male genitalia. Note the depigmentation of the foreskin

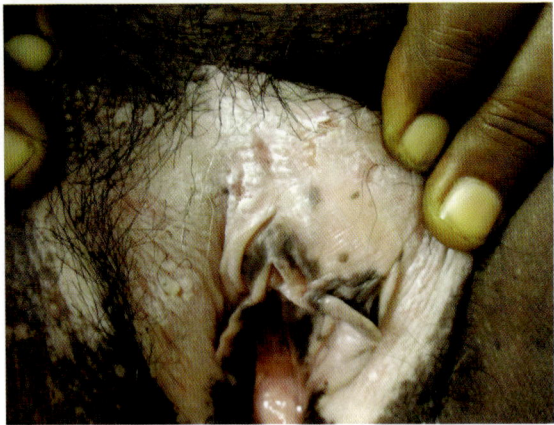

Figure 53: Vitiligo with sclerosis indicating LSA

INTERTRIGO

Intertrigo is an inflammatory condition of skin folds, induced or aggravated by heat, moisture, maceration, friction, and lack of air circulation. Obesity, diabetes, and hyperhidrosis are common risk

Inflammatory Lesions of the Genitalia

factors for intertrigo. Additional factors that predispose individuals to perineal intertrigo include urinary or fecal incontinence, vaginal discharge, or a draining wound.

Intertrigo, frequently, is worsened or colonized by infection. The infective agents may be fungal of which most common is candida, but also may be bacterial. Intertrigo, commonly, affects the axilla, perineum, inframammary creases, and abdominal folds. Diaper dermatitis shows significant overlap with intertrigo. Intertrigo is a common complication of obesity and diabetes. Opposing skin surfaces rub against each other, causing erosions that become inflamed. In the perineal skin, sweat, feces, urine, and vaginal discharge may aggravate intertrigo in both adults and infants. Intertrigo may worsen with heat and humidity or strenuous activity.

Intertrigo usually is chronic with insidious onset of itching, burning, and stinging in skin folds. When acute discomfort is noted, consider secondary infection. Depending on the anatomical site, the presentation may vary (Figs 54 to 57).

Vulva: Vulvitis can occur from erythrasma, plasma cell vulvitis, adult diaper dermatitis, candidal infection, seborrheic dermatitis,

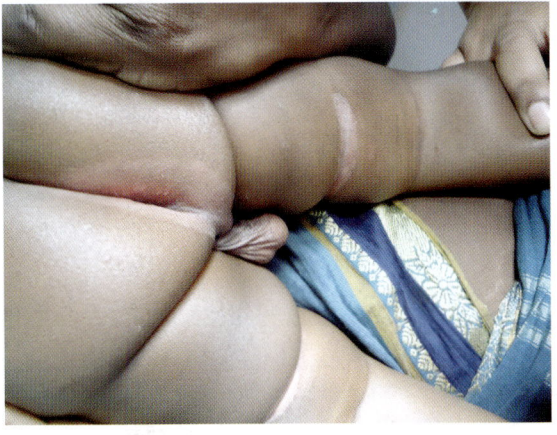

Figure 54: Candidal intertrigo involving the perianal area and the thigh

Genital Dermatoses

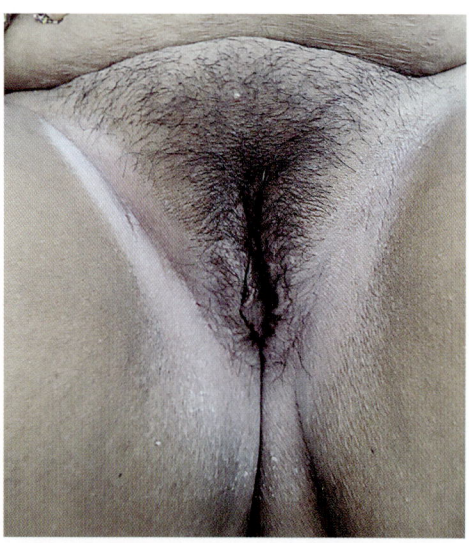

Figure 55: Intertrigo due to constant friction. Note the pustule which is due to secondary infection

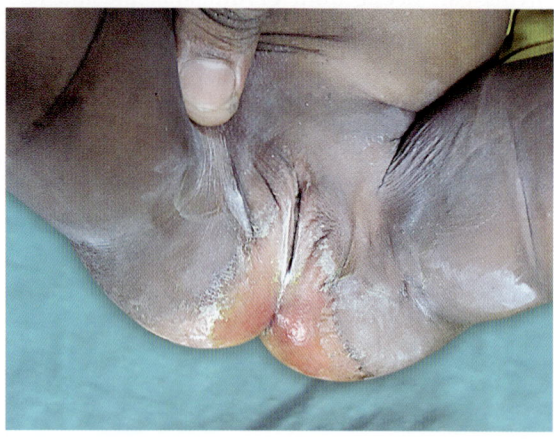

Figure 56: Acrdermatitis enteropathica presenting as erythematous rash of the diaper area

psoriasis, contact dermatitis, or Jaquet "pseudowarts" resulting from chronic maceration.

Inflammatory Lesions of the Genitalia

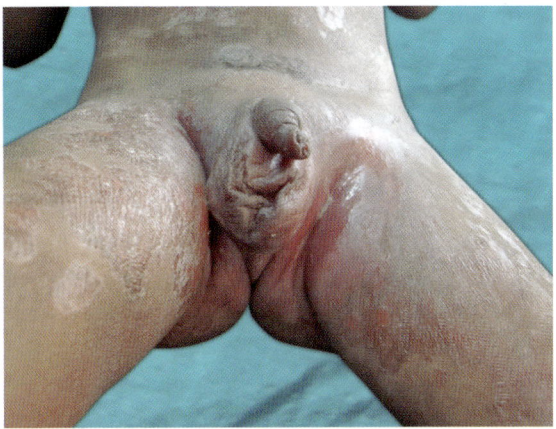

Figure 57: Acrodermatitis enteropathica with intertrigo

Perianal/natal cleft: Consider pruritus ani, candidal infection, contact dermatitis, anal fissures, essential fatty acid deficiency, acrodermatitis enteropathica, extramammary Paget's disease (EMPD), psoriasis, pilonidal cyst, decubitus dermatitis, or baboon syndrome from contact allergy, systemic antibiotics, or hypovitaminosis B.

Crural fold: Alternative diagnoses include inverse psoriasis, candidal infection, adult diaper dermatitis, granuloma inguinale, pemphigus vegetans, benign familial pemphigus (Hailey-Hailey disease), toxic epidermal necrolysis, and EMPD. A form of extensive papulonodular and eroded dermatitis in women appears to be related to overuse of topical preparations, such as vagisil.

Infantile intertrigo: Intertrigo in infants often is synonymous with diaper dermatitis. Exclude seborrheic dermatitis, candidal infection, psoriasis, nutritional abnormalities (biotin deficiency, acrodermatitis enteropathica from zinc deficiency, aminoaciduria related), Letterer-Siwe disease (especially if papular, eroded, or purpuric), granuloma gluteal infantum (from topical corticosteroids), impetigo, cellulitis, cystic fibrosis, congenital syphilis, or hereditary neuroepithelial dysplasia.

Acrodermatitis enteropathica is a rare, inherited form of zinc deficiency, characterized by periorificial and acral dermatitis, alopecia, and diarrhea that can be easily missed as intertrigo, if classical findings are not present.

Treatment

First and foremost is to remove and correct all the precipitating factors and to keep the area dry. Petrolatum, zinc oxide, aluminum acetate, dimethicone alone or in combination can be used to have a barrier effect.

Appropriate antibacterial or antifungal should be used wherever necessary. Zinc supplements are required for treating acrodermatitis enteropathica.

ATROPHIC VULVOVAGINITIS

Vaginal atrophy, also called atrophic vaginitis, is thinning, drying, and inflammation of the vaginal walls due to low levels of estrogen. Vaginal atrophy occurs most often after menopause, but it can also develop during breast-feeding or at any other time when body's estrogen production declines. Postmenopausal women not on estrogen replacement, experience thinning of the vulvar and vaginal epithelium. They may also have thinning of the pubic hair and smoothness and thinning of the vulvar skin. The labia minora and majora lose substance and become more wrinkled; complete resorption of the labia minora occurs in some and may mimic the end stage of lichen sclerosus (Fig. 58).Though patients may be asymptomatic, they complain of sensation of dryness. Some patients complain of dysuria, urgency, and frequency as a result of atrophic urethritis. Dyspareunia is the most common complaint for which patients seek advice. The diagnosis of atrophic vulvovaginitis is by clinical examination and a history of estrogen deficiency. Atrophic vaginitis is suspected when para basal cells and inflammatory cells are seen on wet prep in a symptomatic patient. It is to be remembered that atrophic vulvovaginitis can complicate all vulvovaginal conditions. In the absence of adequate estrogen, the barrier

Inflammatory Lesions of the Genitalia

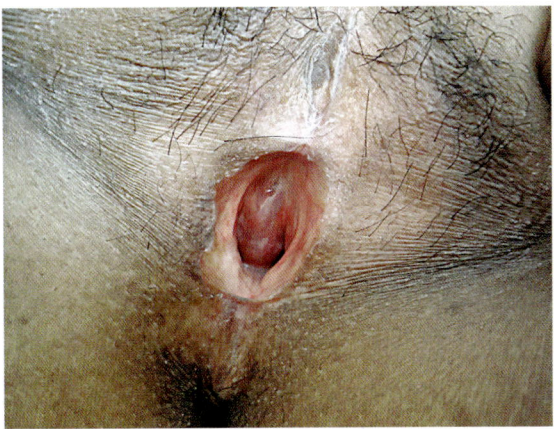

Figure 58: Atrophic vaginitis showing atrophy and erosion of the genital mucosa

functions get weaker and the tissues become more susceptible to irritation. Hygiene practices, sexual activity may further exacerbate the symptoms. This can be further compounded by an already disrupted barrier with lichen sclerosus, lichen planus, even vulval intraepithelial neoplasia.

Treatment

Topical estrogen is to be prescribed. In some women, estrogen can be administered systemically.

CHAPTER 10

Premalignant Lesions of the Genitalia

INTRAEPITHELIAL NEOPLASIA

In situ squamous cell carcinoma (SCC) of the penis, also known as penile intraepithelial neoplasia (PIN), encompasses three clinical variants: Erythroplasia of Queyrat (EQ), Bowen's disease, and bowenoid papulosis (BP). The distinction depends on the anatomic location and clinical presentation of the lesions.

1. Bowen's disease is a clinical presentation of in situ SCC at other sites. EQ represents Bowen's disease on the genital mucosa. The specific etiologic factors remain unclear. Predisposing factors include lack of circumcision, poor hygiene, and chronic infection. Several human papillomavirus (HPV) serotypes have been isolated from this disease, including HPV 8, 16, and 18. Circumcision has been proposed to protect against the development of EQ, possibly secondary to facilitation of better hygiene, less accumulation of smegma, and reduced risk of chronic infections.
2. Erythroplasia of Queyrat presents as a bright-red, well-demarcated, velvety plaque or plaques that involve the glans, coronal sulcus, or prepuce of uncircumcised men. Similar lesions have been described on the vulva.
    Differential diagnoses includes Zoon's balanitis, erosive lichen planus, psoriasis, fixed drug eruption, and seborrheic keratosis.

Histopathology shows features of in situ carcinoma, such as full-thickness epidermal atypia with lack of maturation, nuclear atypia, dyskeratosis, and atypical mitoses. The surface may be eroded or covered with a parakeratotic crust. The underlying dermis typically displays a lymphohistiocytic inflammatory infiltrate. Evidence of tumor invasion into the underlying dermis is absent.

Topical application of 5-fluorouracil cream, imiquimod 5%, laser therapy with neodymium-doped yttrium aluminium garnet (Nd:YAG) or carbon dioxide lasers, cryosurgery, Mohs' micrographic surgery are useful. Excision of the lesion is the definitive treatment.

3. Bowenoid papulosis was first described by Kopf and Bart in 1977. BP is probably a virus-induced epithelial dysplasia mainly associated with HPV type 16, but other types have also been found which include 18, 31, 32, 34, 42, 48, and 51-55. It usually affects sexually active adults with slight female predominance and is more common in smokers. It presents as asymptomatic, flat, hyperpigmented or violaceous papules, few millimeters to several centimeters in size, occurring over the penis, vulva, or perianally (Fig. 1).

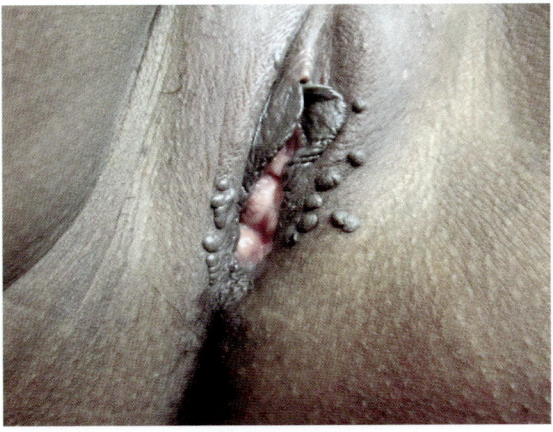

Figure 1: Skin coloured papules of Bowenoid papulosis

Histopathology shows features resembling Bowen's disease. There is crowding and an irregular, wind-blown arrangement of nuclei, many of which are large, hyperchromatic, and pleomorphic. Dyskeratosis, atypical mitoses, and multinucleated keratinocytes are also present. Over time, BP lesions can regress, persists, recur or progress to invasive SCC in some cases. The condition has to be differentiated from genital warts, melanocytic nevi, seborrheic keratosis, lichen planus, Zoon's balanitis, SCC, basal cell carcinoma, and Bowen's disease. Treatment of this condition is mainly by local agents such as 5-fluorouracil, imiquimod, podophylin, and cidofovir. Other modalities include excision, electrocautery, carbon dioxide laser, cryosurgery, photodynamic therapy, and interferon. Retinoid, either topically or systemically, is also effective in treating this condition.

Vulvar intraepithelial neoplasia (VIN) can be graded as VIN1, VIN2, and VIN3, the latter indicating furthest progression toward a true cancer. Usual-type VIN occurs in younger women and is caused by HPV infection. When usual-type VIN changes into invasive SCC, it becomes the basaloid or warty subtypes. The other entity, the differentiated-type VIN tends to occur in older women which is not linked to HPV infection. It can progress to the keratinizing subtype of invasive SCC. The risk of vulvar cancer appears to be slightly increased by LSA, with about 4% of women having LSA later developing vulvar cancer (Fig. 2).

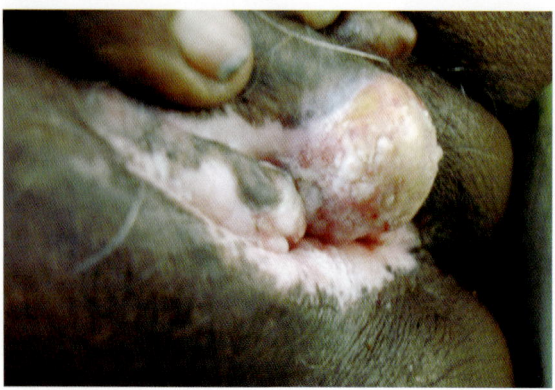

Figure 2: Intra epithelial neoplasia arising from lichen sclerosus et atrophicus

EXTRAMAMMARY PAGET'S DISEASE

Mammary Paget's disease (PD) of the nipple was first described by Sir James Paget in 1874. Extramammary PD (EMPD) was first recognized and reported as a distinct clinical entity by Radcliffe Crocker in 1889. EMPD lesions are typically located in an area of the body, rich in apocrine sweat glands, most commonly the anogenital region and vulva being the most common site. Approximately 25% of the cases of EMPD are associated with an underlying in situ or invasive neoplasm. The cause of primary EMPD is unknown. However, a minority of cases do represent a direct extension of an underlying carcinoma along contiguous epithelium.

It is currently believed, that most cases of vulval EMPD are primary, that is, arising within the epidermis, and very few are associated with cutaneous sweat gland tumors. Vulval EMPD has been described in association with endometrial, endocervical, and vaginal as well as vulval (for example arising within Bartholin's gland), urethral, and bladder neoplasms. Perianal EMPD is rarer than vulvar disease, but is strongly associated with adenocarcinoma of the anus and colorectum. Unlike vulval EMPD, 70-80% of cases of perianal disease arise secondary to invasive malignancy in the anus, rectum, or colon. In common with perianal EMPD, disease of the male genitalia is thought to be more frequently associated with internal malignancy (for example, urethral, bladder, prostatic, and testicular neoplasms) than is vulval EMPD.

Lesions present as moist red oozing plaques, which look like infected eczema or psoriasis, and can present with pruritus and a burning sensation. The disease spreads indolently, by local extension, and metastasis.

The histopathological findings reveal epidermal hyperplasia with atypical Paget's cells in the epidermis, arranged singly or in clusters. Paget's cells are large cells with abundant basophilic or amphophilic, finely granular cytoplasm, which tend to stand out in contrast to the surrounding epithelial cells. On close inspection, the nucleus is usually large, centrally situated, and sometimes contains a prominent nucleolus. Pronounced nuclear atypia and pleomorphism are present. Signet ring cells might be present in small numbers and mitotic figures are frequent. The Paget's cells might be

Genital Dermatoses

dispersed singly or form clusters, glandular structures, or solid nests. There may be infiltration into upper strata of the epidermis, but most cells are concentrated in the lower portion, often being observed in the pilosebaceous apparatus. Cells might be present in sweat gland ducts, leading to confusion as to whether the lesion has arisen within the epidermis or has spread from a local apocrine neoplasm.

The prognosis is excellent in cases that are not associated with an underlying adnexal or visceral tumor.

Treatment is wide excision but conservative vulva-sparing surgery has been recommended in females. Mohs' micrographic surgery has also been used. Cryotherapy, topical 5-fluorouracil, and bleomycin are useful. Topical steroids have been found useful for troublesome pruritus. Radiotherapy is curative in selected cases affecting large areas of the anogenital region.

PSEUDOEPITHELIOMATOUS, KERATOTIC, AND MICACEOUS BALANITIS

Pseudoepitheliomatous, keratotic, and micaceous balanitis (PKMB) was first named and described by Lortat-Jacob and Civatte in 1961. The exact etiology is unknown.

It is mainly seen in elderly over 60 years of age. Though, originally considered to be a benign entity, it has been shown to be capable of invasive growth by Bart and Kopf who considered the lesion to be in intermediate stage between benign hyperplasia and SCC. It has been regarded as a form of pyodermatitis or pseudoepitheliomatous response to infection.

The pathogenesis of PKMB occurs in four stages:

1. Initial plaque stage
2. Late tumor stage
3. Verrucous carcinoma
4. Transformation to SCC and metastasis.

Clinically, it presents as a coronal balanitis, which gradually takes on a silvery-white appearance, and mica like and keratotic horny masses formed on the glans. Sometimes, ulcerations, cracking, and fissuring crusts on the surface of the glans are present. The keratotic scaling is usually micaceous and resembles psoriasis.

Classically, histological examination of these lesions reveals acanthosis, hyperkeratosis, and pseudoepitheliomatous hyperplasia with no cytological atypia.

The treatment of PKMB should be conservative when there is no histological evidence of malignancy. Whenever there is cellular atypia, local surgical excision produces excellent cosmetic and functional results. When frank malignancy is seen, excision with wide margin is the rule.

CHAPTER 11

Malignant Conditions

SQUAMOUS CELL CARCINOMA OF PENIS AND VULVA

Squamous cell carcinoma (SCC) is the most common neoplasm of the genital tract and the penis. The main risk factors for the development of penile SCC are poor hygiene, lack of circumcision, human papillomavirus (HPV) infection, and certain chronic inflammatory skin conditions. Poor hygiene contributes to the development of this tumor through the accumulation of smegma and other irritants in the balanopreputial sulcus. Phimosis interferes with adequate hygiene of the glans, contributes to chronic inflammation, and favors the development of this tumor. A direct relationship has been demonstrated between HPV infection and penile SCC. Both conditions are directly linked to the number of sexual partners. The association with HPV, however, is less common than in cervical cancer, where 95% of patients have this infection. Another risk factor for penile SCC is pseudoepitheliomatous, micaceous, and keratotic balanitis, which affects the glans of elderly, uncircumcised men. It presents as a plaque covered with silver micaceous scales (similar to those seen in psoriasis) that can form a thick keratotic layer. Histologically, its appearance can range from that of simple epithelial hyperkeratosis and hyperplasia, with minimal cytologic atypia, to a lesion mimicking a warty carcinoma.

Malignant Conditions

As occurs with other skin cancers, sustained immunosuppression (e.g., in transplant recipients or patients with human immunodeficiency virus) is closely associated with increased risk of penile SCC and worse prognosis. Finally, penile SCC, like cancer of the bladder and the oral cavity, has been associated with tobacco use.

Clinical Features and Histology

The clinical appearance of invasive penile SCC is highly variable, with manifestations ranging from an erythematous plaque or ulcer to an exophytic or verruciform tumor (Fig. 1). The lesions, which can measure up to several centimeters in diameter, can have a stony hard or friable consistency, and may bleed.

They are more common on the anterior third (glans, balanopreputial sulcus, and/or prepuce). They are found on the shaft of the penis in fewer than 5% of cases.

Several histologic subtypes have been identified on the basis of architectural and cytologic features. Keratinizing, or usual SCCs are the most common forms of invasive penile SCC and account for 50–60% of all cases; they generally follow an infiltrative growth pattern

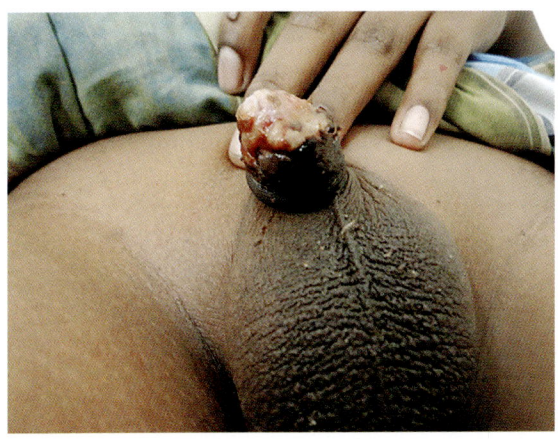

Figure 1: Invasive penile SCC with exophytic tumour involving glans and shaft of penis

Genital Dermatoses

and can be well or poorly differentiated. Verrucous penile SCC (8–10% of the cases) is architecturally similar to a wart and follows an expansive growth pattern. Basaloid penile SCC (4–6% of the cases) is characterized by the presence of nests of clearly basaloid cells with an infiltrating pattern and peripheral palisading, while warty penile SCC (6–10% of the cases) resembles a wart and has easily identifiable cytopathic changes and larger cells. Verrucous and warty types have the best prognosis; basaloid, sarcomatoid, and undifferentiated usual tumors are all associated with a high risk of dissemination.

TNM classification of penile SCC according to the European Association of Urologists Guidelines on Penile Cancer 2009 is as follows:

T: Primary tumor
TX: Primary tumor cannot be assessed
T0: No evidence of primary tumor
Ta: Noninvasive verrucous carcinoma
T1: Tumor invades subepithelial connective tissue
T1a: No lymphovascular invasion and the tumor is well differentiated or moderately differentiated (T1-G1/G2)
T1b: Lymphovascular invasion and the tumor is poorly differentiated or undifferentiated (T1-G3/G4)
T2: Tumor invades corpus spongiosum or corpora cavernosa
T3: Tumor invades urethra
T4: Tumor invades other adjacent structures.
N: Regional lymph nodes (p: pathologic classification)
NX: Regional lymph nodes cannot be assessed
N0: No palpable or visibly-enlarged inguinal lymph nodes
N1: Palpable mobile unilateral inguinal lymph node
N2: Palpable mobile multiple or bilateral inguinal lymph nodes
N3: Fixed inguinal nodal mass or pelvic lymphadenopathy—unilateral or bilateral.
M: Distant metastasis
M0: No distant metastasis
M1: Lymph node metastasis outside the true pelvis in addition to visceral sites.

Treatment

The mainstay treatment for invasive penile SCC is surgical resection of the primary tumor with margins of 5–10 mm. The goal of treatment is to eliminate the disease, and where possible, to preserve urinary and sexual function. Wide circumcision is the treatment of choice when the prepuce is involved; for more invasive tumors, glansectomy or partial penectomy (depending on the size of the tumor) should be considered. Total penectomy is an option, when the tumor is located on the shaft of the penis or is poorly differentiated. Radiotherapy of the primary tumor is an option in T1 or T2 tumors measuring less than 4 cm in diameter, and is associated with 5-year cure rates of 70–90%.

Penile SCC is a preventable disease. Patients with phimosis that prevents adequate exploration and good glans hygiene should be circumcised. Because HPV infection, particularly HPV-16 infection, is a key factor in the etiology of certain types of penile SCC, HPV vaccines may have beneficial effects, if administered to boys before they become sexually active.

Squamous cell carcinoma is the most common vulvar malignancy. It can occur commonly in elderly women with a background of a chronic dermatoses like lichen sclerosus et atrophicus or lichen planus (Figs 2 and 3), or can occur in younger women in association with intraepithelial neoplasia associated with oncogenic-type HPV infection. Vulvar SCC is classified histologically into three types: keratinizing, basaloid, and warty carcinomas. Lypmhatics are affected and distant metastasis occurs. Surgical excision is recommended and has to be individualized. In those with inoperable tumors, radiotherapy is preferred.

BASAL CELL CARCINOMA

Basal cell carcinoma (BCC) occurs in patients after the fifth decade of life. Advancing age and local trauma may contribute to the pathogenesis of BCC at these sites. At presentation, the lesion is

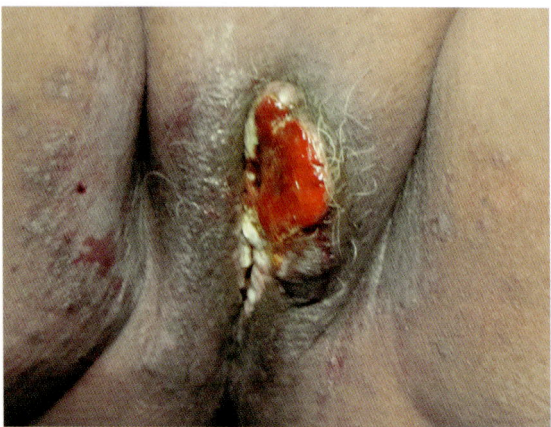

Figure 2: SCC arising from lichen sclerosus et atrophicus

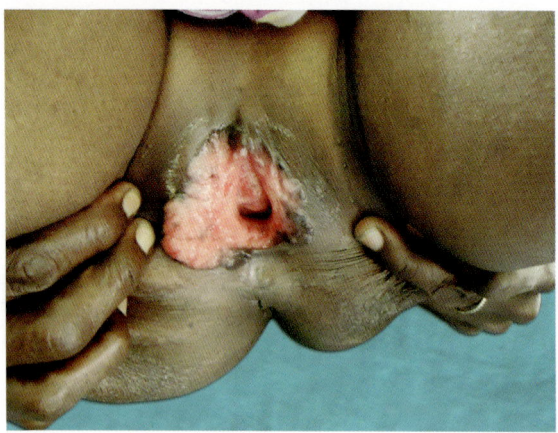

Figure 3: SCC from lichen planus. Note the violaceous margin

usually large in size; pigmented, and is eroded or ulcerated in about one-third of patients. The most frequent site is the labia majora. Biopsy reveals aggregates of basaloid cells with peripheral palisading and clefts between the aggregates and the stroma. Excision is the treatment of choice.

MALIGNANT MELANOMA

Melanomas of the penis and vulva are rare and comprise about 1% and 4–10% of all malignancies at these sites, respectively, in Caucasians. They are rarer in the scrotum. It usually presents as a pigmented macule or nodule, which may ulcerate or bleed. Biopsy of the lesion reveals a poorly circumscribed lesion with typical melanocytes within the epidermis and in irregular aggregates in the dermis that vary in size and pigmentation. The melanocytes have large nuclei with prominent nucleoli and do not diminish in size with descent into the dermis.

Wide local excision with a clear margin is the treatment of choice. Surgical therapy may be combined with chemotherapy.

CHAPTER 12

Other Diseases of the Genitalia

Other rare tumors are Kaposi sarcoma, fibrosarcoma, leiomyosarcoma, malignant fibrous histiocytoma, epithelioid sarcoma, liposarcoma, and spindle cell sarcoma. Primary adenocarcinoma of the vulva is exceedingly rare.

PEYRONIE'S DISEASE

Peyronie's disease also known as induratio penis plastic or chronic inflammation of the tunica albuginea (CITA), is a connective tissue disorder involving the growth of fibrous plaques in the soft tissue of the penis affecting 5% of men (Fig. 1). Specifically, scar tissue forms in the tunica albuginea, the thick sheath of tissue surrounding the corpora cavernosa causing pain, abnormal curvature, erectile dysfunction, indentation, loss of girth, and shortening. Variety of treatments have been used, but none have been especially effective.

The pathogenesis of peyronie's disease is not clearly understood, but the current paradigm suggests that it is a wound-healing disorder occurring in a genetically susceptible individual whose tunica albuginea responds inappropriately to an inciting event, most commonly trauma, with a proliferative fibrotic reaction resulting in an exuberant, inelastic scar that does not resolve. Of note, only 25–30% of men presenting with peyronie's disease recall a traumatic event, suggesting that the high pressures that occur within the penis

Other Diseases of the Genitalia

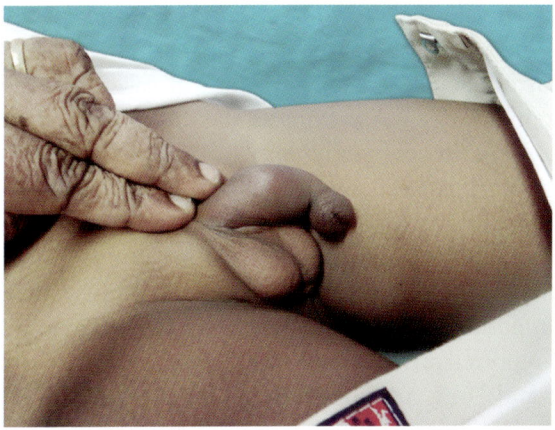

Figure 1: Peyronie's disease showing abnormal curvature of penis

during coitus may create forces, which the tunic cannot withstand, resulting in a silent microfracture. Discussion of the putative etiologic and pathological factors causing peyronie's disease is beyond the scope of this book, except to note that it appears that the peyronie's disease plaque does not resolve due to absent or malfunctioning metalloproteinases and/or elevated levels of tissue inhibitors of metalloproteinases (TIMPs), resulting in a scar which does not undergo normal remodeling.

A certain degree of curvature of the penis is considered normal, as many men are born with this benign condition, commonly referred to as congenital curvature.

The disease may cause pain, hardened, big, cord-like lesions, or abnormal curvature of the penis (Fig. 1), when erect due to CITA. Although the popular conception of peyronie's disease is that it always involves curvature of the penis, the scar tissue sometimes causes divots or indentations rather than curvature. The condition may also make sexual intercourse painful and/or difficult.

Injection therapy has also been used for many years, starting with intralesional steroid injection. The rationale here is reasonable, as steroids have anti-inflammatory and possibly antifibrotic properties, but no real benefit with respect to objective measures has ever been published, and side effects from repeated exposure to steroids have been reported. Intralesional verapamil makes scientific sense, as studies have shown decreased peyronie's disease-derived fibroblast proliferation and decreased extracellular matrix production *in vitro*. A recent animal model study demonstrated reduction of cellular proliferation, decreased myofibroblast activity, and increased metalloproteinase activity when verapamil was exposed to peyronie's disease plaque-derived fibroblasts in tissue culture.

Interferon 2β is considered a biological modifier that may have similar properties to verapamil. Intralesional collagenase has been used and reported on since the early 1980s. It was recently submitted for Food and Drug Administration (FDA) approval in the United States.

With respect to topical therapy, the International Consultation concluded that "as there are no independent controlled trials and no evidence of adequate levels within the tunica albuginea , no recommendation is possible for topical verapamil."

Vacuum therapy has been touted as a potential treatment for peyronie's disease.

PENILE HORN

Cornu cutaneum or the cutaneous horn is a peculiar type of benign neoplasm, showing horn-like projection on the skin. Although the cutaneous horn may develop over a normal skin, these more often develop over some pre-existing skin conditions like warts, keratoses, nevi, trauma, burns, lupus vulgaris, and even on an epithelioma. In the normal process of keratinization, the dead keratin is being gradually cast off as dust. If this keratin continues to stick on, the result is a horn which represents marked cohesiveness of the keratin. Since the horn represents an erroneous epithelial growth, it may sometimes be complicated with malignancy.

The etiology of penile horns is uncertain, although they are often found in association with warts, phimosis, nevi, and in areas afflicted by trauma. Malignant change should be suspected in a rapidly growing lesion. Microscopically, a cutaneous horn shows marked hyperkeratosis, acanthosis, dyskeratosis, papillomatosis, and chronic inflammatory infiltration of the adjacent dermis.

Treatment options include wide surgical excision with careful histological examination to exclude a focus of malignancy. If malignancy is present in a penile cutaneous horn, the treatment involves partial penectomy with or without regional lymph node dissection. Therapy with carbon dioxide or neodymium yttrium aluminium garnet (Nd:YAG) laser is used for patients who refuse surgery. While preliminary studies with laser are encouraging, partial penectomy remains the gold standard.

SCROTAL CALCINOSIS

Scrotal calcinosis (SC) is characterized by calcific deposits with surrounding foreign body type granulomatous inflammation in the scrotal skin. This benign scrotal lesion, presenting as asymptomatic firm to hard nodules (Fig. 2) though commonly occurs between third and fourth decades of life, can affect both adult and pediatric age groups with age range between 9 and 85 years reported in the literature. SC is more common in dark-colored race and affects mainly males, but similar lesions (vulvar calcinosis) has been reported in females.

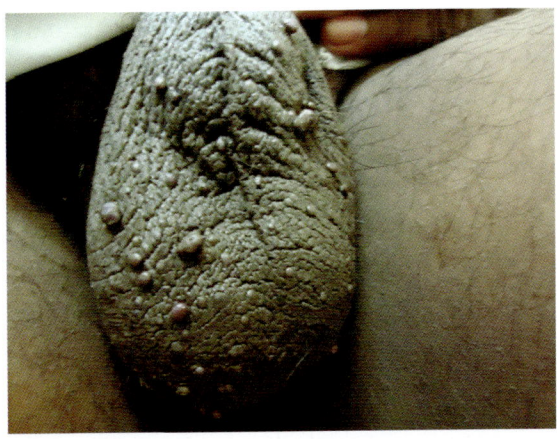

Figure 2: Multiple scrotal cyst that eventually calcify

The pathogenesis of SC is unclear and controversy exists as to whether the disease is idiopathic or the result of dystrophic calcification of pre-existing structures, including epidermal cyst, eccrine epithelial cyst, and degenerated dartos muscle. The calcification of pre-existent epidermal cysts is suggested by many authors as a possible pathogenesis. Calcification of epidermal cysts occurs after an inflammatory reaction that triggers a degenerative process and eventually leads to the resorption of the cyst walls and the loss of their epithelial lining. However, some researchers found that dystrophic calcification of the dartos muscle was the basis of SC, and they suggested that degeneration and necrosis of the dartos muscle are the initial events in the pathogenesis of disease. Ito and colleagues proposed that SC originates from eccrine epithelial cysts and the pathogenic mechanism seems to be the excessive discharge and accumulation of material debris in the lumina. This eccrine origin was discovered via an immunohistochemical study using antibodies against carcinoembryonic antigen, epithelial membrane antigen, and gross cystic disease fluid protein.

The main reason patient seek intervention is because of cosmetic concern. Patient with intense pruritus or ulceration will require surgical intervention. Smaller lesions are amenable to the novel pinch-punch excision. Larger lesions may require wide excision and direct closure can be achieved in most patients as shown in our index case. Extensive disease, involving the whole scrotum or florid recurrent disease, will require complex scrotal reconstruction.

Even though SC is a benign condition, it is important to let patient know about the possibility of recurrence. Recurrence may be due to left-over microscopic foci of calcification.

FOURNIER'S GANGRENE

Fournier's gangrene (FG) is a fulminant form of infective necrotizing fasciitis of the perineal, genital, or perianal regions, which commonly affects men, but can also occur in women and children. Even though this clinical entity is eponymously credited to the Parisian venereologist Jean Alfred Fournier, who described it as a fulminant gangrene of the penis and scrotum in young men, Baurienne in 1764 and Avicenna in 1877 had described the same disease earlier. Over the years, many terms have been used to describe this clinical condition including idiopathic gangrene of the scrotum, periurethral phlegmon, streptococcal scrotal gangrene, phagedena, and synergistic necrotizing cellulitis.

Initially, FG was defined as an idiopathic entity, but diligent search will show the source of infection in the vast majority of cases, as either perineal or genital skin infections. Anorectal or urogenital and perineal trauma, including pelvic and perineal injury or pelvic interventions are other causes of FG. The most common foci include the gastrointestinal tract (30-50%), followed by the genitourinary tract (20-40%), and cutaneous injuries (20%). Comorbid systemic disorders are being identified more and more in patients with FG, the most common being diabetes mellitus and alcohol misuse.

In FG, suppurative bacterial infection results in microthrombosis of the small subcutaneous vessels leading to the development of gangrene of the overlying skin. Cultures from the wounds commonly show polymicrobial infections by aerobes and anaerobes, which include coliforms, *Klebsiella, Streptococci, Staphylococci, Clostridia, Bacteroids,* and *Corynebacteria.* The synergistic activity of aerobes and anaerobes lead to the production of various exotoxins and enzymes like collagenase, heparinase, hyaluronidase, streptokinase, and streptodornase, which aid in tissue destruction and spread of infection. The platelet aggregation and complement fixation induced by the aerobes and the heparinase and collagenase produced by the anaerobes lead to microvascular thrombosis and dermal necrosis. In addition, the phagocytic activity is impaired in the necrotic tissue, aiding in further spread of the infection.

Fournier's gangrene shows vast heterogeneity in clinical presentation, from insidious onset and slow progression to rapid onset and fulminant course, the latter being the more common presentation. The infection commonly starts as a cellulitis adjacent to the portal of entry, depending on the source of infection, commonly in the perineum or perianal region. The local signs and symptoms are usually dramatic with significant pain and swelling. The patient also has pronounced systemic signs; usually out of proportion to the local extent of the disease. Crepitus of the inflamed tissues is a common feature because of the presence of gas-forming organisms. As the subcutaneous inflammation worsens, necrotic patches start appearing over the overlying skin and progress to extensive necrosis. Unless aggressively treated, the patient can rapidly progress to sepsis with multiple-organ failure, the common cause of death in these patients. The spread of infection is along the facial planes and is usually limited by the attachment of the Colles' fascia in the perineum. Infection can spread to involve the scrotum, penis, and can spread up the anterior abdominal wall, up to the clavicle. The testes are usually spared as their blood supply originates intra-abdominally. Involvement of the testis suggests retroperitoneal origin or spread of infection. Urogenital infections travel posteriorly along the Bucks and Dartos fascia to involve the Colles' fascia, but are limited from the anal margin by the attachment of the Colles' fascia to the perineal body. In contrast, anorectal sources of infection usually start perianaly and this variation in initial clinical presentation can serve as a guide to localizing the foci of infection.

CUTANEOUS LYMPHANGIECTASIA

Cutaneous lymphangiectasia is also called as acquired lymphangioma. It is a benign cutaneous disorder involving the dermal and subcutaneous lymphatic channels. Cutaneous lymphangiectasias arise due to the obstruction of the lymphatics secondary and are not true neoplasms or hamartomas. Damage to the lymphatics can result from radiation, surgery, trauma, keloid, scrofuloderma, pregnancy, scleroderma, neoplasia, or infections such as filariasis, tuberculosis, recurrent erysipelas, and lymphogranuloma venereum. Vulval lymphangiectasia is a rare disease and is usually reported following surgery/radiotherapy for carcinoma of the cervix or vulva, tubercular inguinal lymphadenitis, or Crohn's disease of the vulva. Vulvar lymphangiectasia can be asymptomatic, pruritic, burning, or painful, clinically characterized by vulval edema, studded with thin-walled translucent vesicles sometimes containing serosanguineous fluid, which at a later stage, become firm and hyperkeratotic (Figs 3 to 5). There can be frequent episodes of secondary infection. Histologically, dilated lymphatic channels are present in the superficial and mid-dermis; few dilated

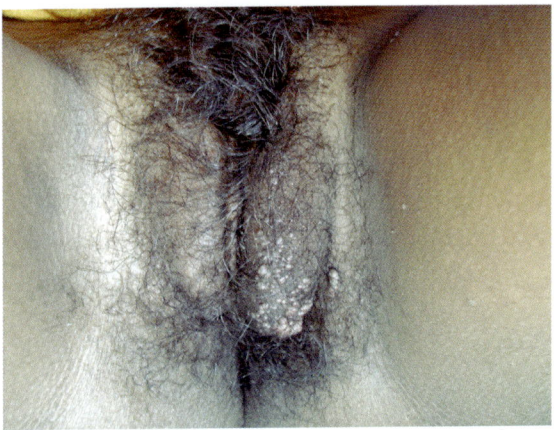

Figure 3: Lymphangiectasia in a pregnant women

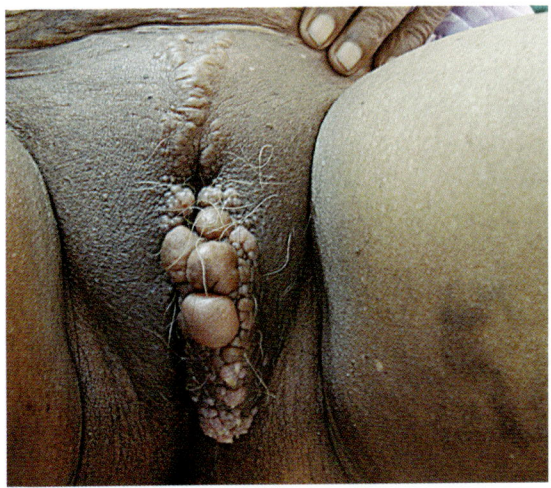

Figure 4: Lymphangiectasia in a women following radiotherapy

Genital Dermatoses

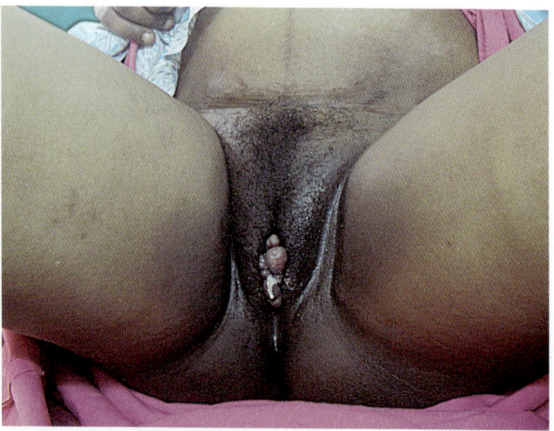

Figure 5: Vulval oedema of pregnancy giving raise to lymphangiectasia

lymphatics are seen in the deep dermis. The overlying epidermis may display varying degrees of hyperkeratosis, acanthosis, and papillomatosis, and it may appear to enclose the ectatic lymphatic channels. These dilated lymphatic channels may contain scattered lymphocytes and red blood cells, imparting a purplish tinge to the lesion. Vulvar lymphangiectasia has to be distinguished from lymphangioma circumscriptum (LC). LC is a congenitally derived hamartoma with early onset of the lesions.

Treatment

It is self-limiting in conditions like pregnancy. Treatment is aimed at reduction of underlying lymphedema and control of infection. In cases where infection is responsible, treatment should be instituted as early as possible to lessen the damage to the lymphatics. Daily compression bandage can help in some patients, though it is difficult in sites like vulva. Excisional surgery, carbon dioxide laser, cryotherapy, electrocoagulation, and sclerozing agent injection are the modalities of therapy.

BARTHOLIN'S GLAND DISEASES

Bartholin's glands cysts and abscesses in women are common problem during the reproductive age. Approximately, 1–2% of women develop a Bartholin's cyst at some time in life. They are exceedingly rare before puberty. Bartholin's gland enlargement in patients older than 40 years is rare and should be subjected for histological study to rule out other diseases. Bartholin's gland abscess is a rarity in infants and children (Fig. 6), however, it has been reported even in neonates and infants as young as three months old.

Cysts and abscesses are often clinically distinguishable. Obstruction usually secondary to nonspecific inflammation or trauma of the ostium of the duct leads to the formation of Bartholin's cysts leading to distension of the gland or duct with fluid. The cyst is 1–3 cm in diameter and usually asymptomatic, although larger cysts may be associated with pain and dyspareunia. Infection of the cyst or the gland leads to the development of Bartholin's abscesses which usually presents with acute, rapidly progressive vulvar pain associated with sudden increase in the existing swelling of the cyst. Culture of the aspirate demonstrate a polymicrobial cause.

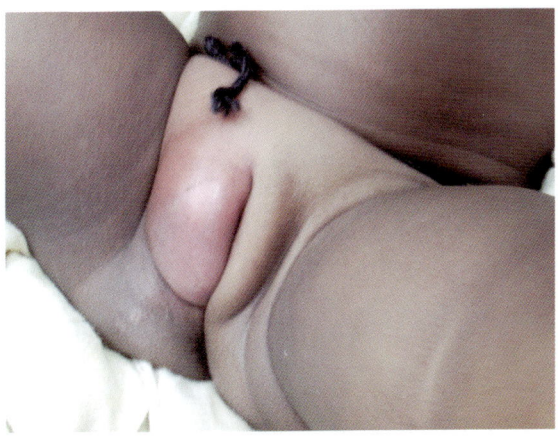

Figure 6: Bartholin abscess in an infant

Swelling of the genitals can occur due to many causes that also includes other causes of genital swelling like infection, insect bite, venous insufficiency, allergic reaction, blunt trauma, cellulitis, C1esterase deficiency, hereditary and acquired angioedema, as part of generalized edema should be excluded in early cases of Bartholin's gland abscess.

Very rarely, adenocarcinoma can arise from the Bartholin's glands, accounting for 1–2% of all vulvar malignancies. Postmenopausal woman with an asymptomatic enlargement of the gland should be followed up, and biopsy should be done in case of suspicion.

Treatment

Uncomplicated, asymptomatic cyst may be advised sitz bath. Sitz baths for several days may promote improvement with resolution. Spontaneous rupture can happen resulting in resolution of the cyst.

A Bartholin's abscess requires incision and drainage using adequate anesthesia aiming to allow complete drainage and to prevent rapid reaccumulation of fluid.

Bartholin's gland carcinoma should be managed by specialists, with surgery and chemoradiotherapy using external-beam radiation therapy (EBRT), high-dose-rate interstitial brachytherapy (HDR-ISBT) boost as the case may be.

Marsupialization is a procedure where wide incision of the mass is followed by suturing the inner edge to the external mucosa, used in persons with recurrent abscesses.

Excision of the Bartholin's gland and surrounding tissue is usually not indicated in the treatment of abscess except to treat malignancy.

Silver nitrate ablation, carbon dioxide laser therapy and, alcohol sclerotherapy give promising results in the treatment for both simple cysts and abscesses.

BENIGN LESIONS OF THE GENITAL SKIN

Benign neoplasms of the vagina are uncommon. The frequency of benign lesions ranges from rare to very rare. Neoplasms that may develop in other locations within the genital tract may also be found in the vagina. Most vaginal tumors produce no symptoms until significant size is reached. Symptoms and signs may include a sensation of pressure, dyspareunia, obstruction of the vagina or urethra, or vaginal bleeding. However, most lesions will be detected during a routine exam in the asymptomatic patient. Vaginal neoplasms may be divided into cystic or solid lesions and a third category best described as related conditions. As is true for any neoplasm, biopsy provides a definitive diagnosis.

Cystic tumours include: Gartner's duct cyst, paramesonephric duct cyst, inclusion cyst, and endometriosis. Leiomyoma, fibroepithelial polyp, hemangiopericytoma, neurofibromas, mixed cell tumors, granular cell myoblastoma, myxoma, rhabdomyoma, and benign cystic teratoma are rare neoplasms found in the vagina. Excisional biopsy is required to make the diagnosis. The genital skin can also develop tumours seen elsewhere in the body.

Benign scrotal masses are not uncommon. These may include: hematocele, hydrocele, spermatocele, or varicocele. Scrotal masses can be caused by inguinal hernia, epididymitis, injury, testicular torsion, and tumors like angiolymphoid hyperplasia with eosinophilia can affect the scrotum and genital skin.

Common benign diseases seen in the vulval region as an isolated entity or as part of the widespread disease include congenital melanocytic nevus, epidermal nevus, and neurofibromatosis (Figs. 7 to 10). Vascular lesions like hemangioma and angiolymphoid

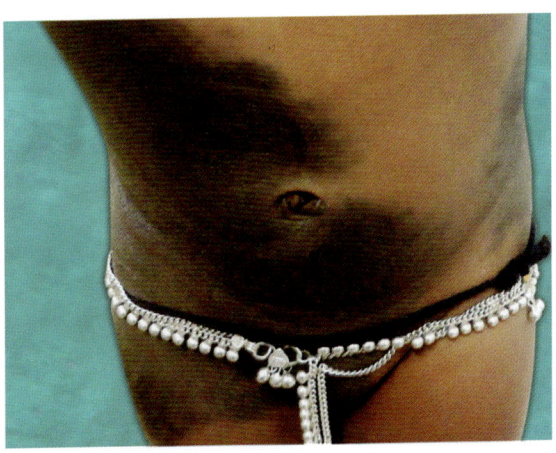

Figure 7: Congenital melanocytic nevus in a child

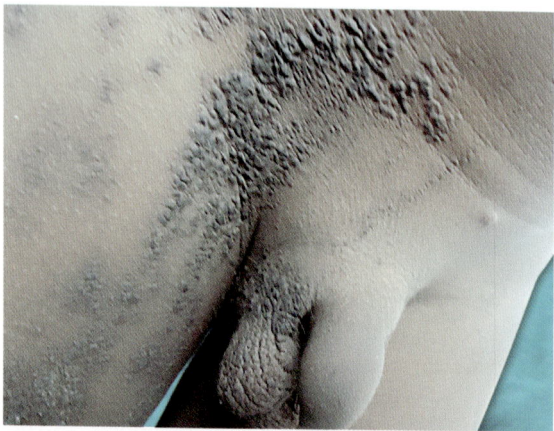

Figure 8: Genital skin involvement in epidermal nevus

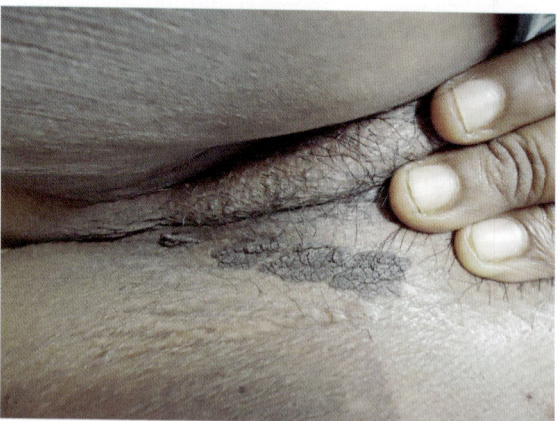

Figure 9: Localised Epidermal nevus involving genital skin

hyperplasia with eosinophilia though rare, have been reported to occur over vulva (Figs 11 and 12). Incontinentia pigmenti and transient neonatal pustular melanosis are common in the neonatal

Other Diseases of the Genitalia

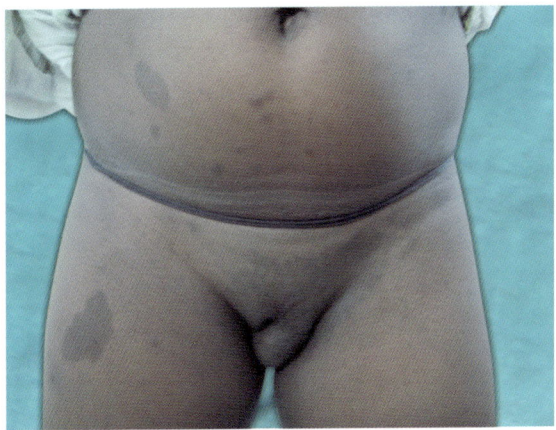

Figure 10: Neurofibromatosis, showing cafe au lait macule and genital involvement

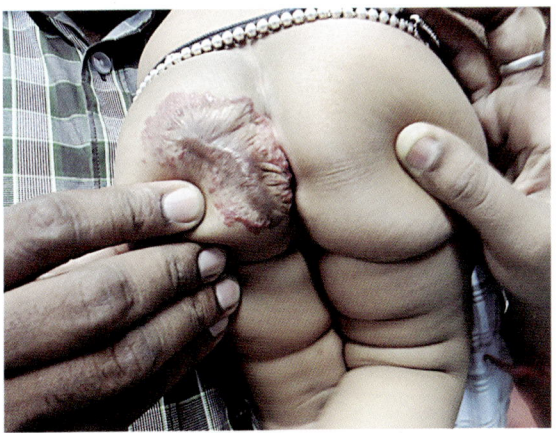

Figure 11: Infantile haemangioma of the perianal and gluteal skin

age group to affect the genital skin (Figs 13 and 14). Giant soft fibroma is rare, but not uncommon tumor of the genital skin. Due to the size and friction, they can lead to mechanical discomfort.

Genital Dermatoses

Frequent secondary infection will warrant excision of the tumor either by cauterization if the pedicle is small or by surgery (Fig. 15).

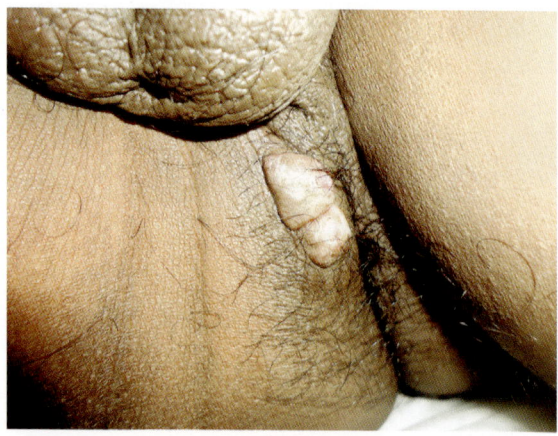

Figure 12: Angiolymphoid hyperplasia of the genital skin

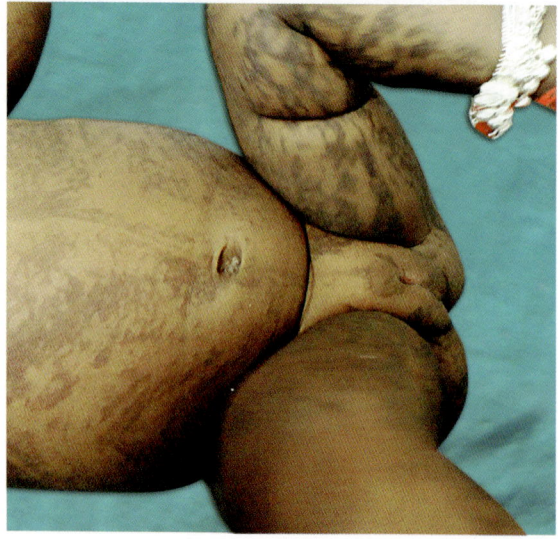

Figure 13: Incontenentia pigmenti involving the genital skin

Other Diseases of the Genitalia

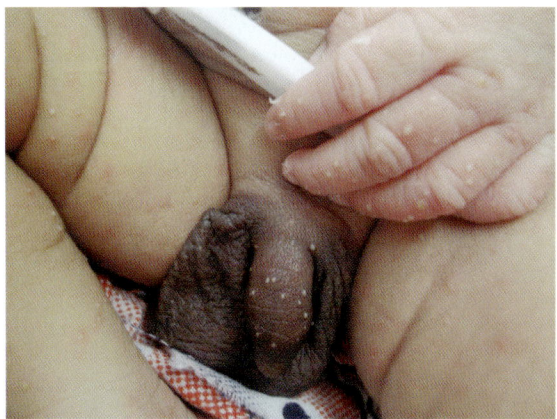

Figure 14: Superficial pustules of transient neonatal pustular melanosis in a newborn

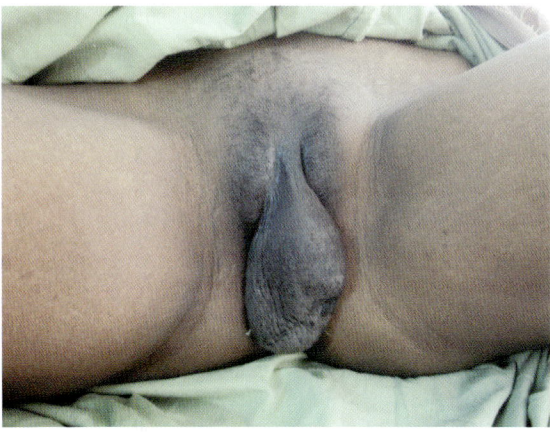

Figure 15: Soft fibroma from the labia majora

CHAPTER 13

Genital Pain Syndrome

The complaint of burning seems more common on mucous membranes than on keratinized epithelium, and pruritus is reported to occur more frequently on gential mucosa than on oral mucosa.

Chronic genital pain, burning or the sensation of irritation in the absence of obvious physical findings is an occasional but debilitating syndrome. Vulvodynia (burning of the vulva) is far more common that scrotodynia or penile pain. Complaints of vulval pain are becoming much more common. The term "vulvodynia" has been applied to a group of symptoms characterized by chronic and often unremitting pain, burning, stinging or rawness of the vulval area. Pruritus is absent. Examination shows neither signs of primary disease nor secondary changes associated with rubbing or scratching. Adult age groups are involved and many patients will indicate the precise localization of symptoms. Vulvodynia is often multifactorial. Vast majority of women are extremely depressed and experience major disruption in their sexual functioning. It is generally not believed to result primarily from psychosexual dysfunction. Since the cause of this syndrome is unknown, treatment is empirical and should be as conservative as possible.

VULVODYNIA

The subtypes of vulvodynia are mentioned below.

Cyclic Vulvovaginitis (Cyclic Vulvitis)

Episodic vulvodynia with freedom from symptoms between recurrences is typical of cyclic vulvovaginitis. It is characterized by intermittent pruritus and burning that may be associated with erythema or the sensation of swelling. Symptoms vary with the menstrual cycle and are worsened after coitus. It is usually seen in premenopausal woman or a woman on estrogen-replacement therapy. These patients have redness and inflammation at the introitus, and the skin splits easily, probably as a result of underlying edema. Vaginal discharge is rare. There is history of frequent candidal infection and frequent use of antibiotics for sinus conditions, urinary tract infection or acne. The speculation is that this condition may be associated with changes in the vaginal ecosystem, because many patients report recurrence of symptoms at the time of menses or after intercourse.

Vulvar Vestibulitis Syndrome

The vestibule is the inner portion of the vulva. It extends from the hymenal ring laterally to the Hart's line (the junction of the keratinized skin and mucosa) on the inner surface of the labia minora, anteriorly to and includes the frenulum of the clitoris and posteriorly down to and includes the fourchette. This marks the beginning of vulvovaginal mucous membrane. This is the only portion of the female genital tract that is derived from endoderm. It is covered with epithelium that is not keratinized, and has characteristics that lie between mucous membrane and skin. It has all the sensitivity of mucous membrane and little of the resistance of skin. Into this space open the major vestibular glands (Bartholin's, Skene's, and periurethral) and minor vestibular glands, which may number a few to many.

The term vulvar vestibulitis syndrome (VVS) is applied to a constellation of symptoms and signs consisting of pain on penile entry (introital dyspareunia), findings confined to focal erythema within the vulvar vestibule, and exquisite tenderness on light palpation of erythematous areas that involve and limited to the vulvar vestibule. In those, who are not sexually active, complaints range from pain on touching the vulvar vestibule, to pain on tampon insertion, on prolonged sitting, on riding a bicycle, on crossing the legs or wearing tight jeans. Except for these activities, patients are asymptomatic. The pain of VVS is typically chronic and continuous. Clinical findings are meager and confine to the vulvar vestibule. There is always erythema. VVS is one of the recognized subsets of vulvodynia. It is one of the most disabling subtypes of vulvodynia and is the most difficult to treat. The term VVS must be reserved for those patients whose symptoms are more than 6 months duration. Pain is not spontaneous; it is elicited by pressure on the erythematous areas within the vulvar vestibule.

The cause of VVS is unknown. The great majority of cases are idiopathic. According to one recent theory, the alkaline urine from dietary oxalate irritates the genital skin and inflames the vestibular glands. Hence, the patients are advised to take low-oxalate diet (e.g., asparagus, chocolate, and many green leafy vegetables) and to take calcium citrate to bind the dietary oxalates. It has been found to be associated with subclinical human papillomavirus (HPV) infection, chronic recurrent candidiasis, and persistent alteration of vaginal pH above or below normal pH which varies from 4.0 to 4.5 and therapy for some of these conditions sometimes leads to amelioration of the symptoms. There are also some reports of development of VVS after the disappearance of acute vulvitis due to chemical therapeutic agents and after laser therapy. Many believe that this syndrome is a form of reflex sympathetic dystrophy. Patients who describe episodic vestibulitis with symptom-free intervals, even if they are only occasional, have a better prognosis for recovery. Remissions have occurred spontaneously and with conservative therapy.

SCROTODYNIA AND PENILODYNIA

Scrotum or penis, usually glans penis, burns often. Patients describe of significant erythema, but on examination there is very little inflammation. Because of the rarity of this condition (scrotodynia), it is poorly understood. There is very little published information regarding causes and therapy. Some experienced clinicians feel that it is usually a manifestation of psychosexual dysfunction.

Chronic Perianal Pain and the "Perianal Syndrome"

Sensations of pain without any evident organic cause localized to the anogential region have been described under a number of names.

- Proctalgia fugax, which affects young adult males, occurs chiefly at night in the form of a sudden cramp-like pain and resolves in a few minutes
- "Coccygodynia descending perineum pain" and "chronic idiopathic anal pain" affects chiefly females. Pain is dull and throbbing and is often precipitated by sitting. Treatment is disappointing.

Dermatologists sometimes may be confronted by a problem in which the patient complains of short-lived episodes of intense burning limited to perineum or occasionally scrotum, which may be accompanied by sweating. The attacks occur without any warning but sometimes may be brought about by a full rectum. The patients usually tend to be under stress, and the skin is entirely normal in these conditions.

Mechanism is unknown. Cholinergic may be suggested because of relief from propantheline. The group may also fall into the group of "dermatological nondiseases". Similar condition has been reported in children suffering from intrafamilial stresses.

When we begin wondering about these pain syndromes, we will hear and see other areas of the body involved as pain and itch sensation are carried on the same unmyelinated type C nerve fibers.

Treatment

In VVS, application of 5% xylocaine ointment, 15–30 minutes prior to intercourse and the use of sore protective coating (e.g. petroleum jelly etc.) are useful.

In dysesthetic vulvodynia, topical 5% lidocaine ointment applied as often as the patients wish is often helpful.

In some cases of cyclic vulvovaginitis, intermittent douching with sodium bicarbonate or vinegar may be beneficial.

There are anecdotal reports that topical steroids and capsaicin offer temporary relief. Some patients experience some relief from cold applications.

Antidepressants are used widely to treat symptoms other than depression, many of which fit into a general category of pain. Tricyclic antidepressants, such as amitriptyline, clomipramine, doxepin, and imipramine are effective in several of these conditions. They have serotonergic, noradrenergic, anticholinergic, and antihistaminic properties. Their analgesic effect differs from their antidepressant effect, in that way that lower dose is sufficient.

Consistent long-term anticandidal therapy seems to be successful treatment strategy in cyclic vulvovaginitis.

In VVS, there are anecdotal reports of temporary relief of pain from pudendal and epidural nerve block, with or without the addition of systemic steroids.

Patients with VVS, who are recalcitrant to conservative measures, sometimes improve with local interferon-α injections and surgical excision of the painful area with advancement of vaginal mucosa.

In VVS, at times, various forms of laser therapy have been used successfully, but therapy carries the risk of worsening the condition.

There is some evidence that hormone replacement may help in a few postmenopausal patients.

Biofeedback, stress reduction techniques, acupuncture, transepidermal nerve stimulation, and muscle relaxation techniques, which have been tried in other pain conditions, can be evaluated as alternative therapies.

Supportive psychotherapy might be indicated for some patients, in whom chronic pain leads to depression, to help them cope with this problem.

Bibliography

1. Alikhan A, Lynch PJ, Eisen DB. Hidradenitis suppurativa: A comprehensive review. J Am Acad Dermatol. 2009;60(4):539-61.
2. An T, Ferenczy A, Wilens SL, Melicow M. Observations on the formation of Michaelis-Gutmann bodies. Hum Pathol. 1974;5(6):753-8.
3. Cameron CE. Identification of a Treponema pallidum laminin-binding protein. Infect Immun. 2003;71(5):2525-33.
4. Centers for Disease Control and Prevention Website, Sexually transmitted disease guidelines. [online] Available from: http://www.cdc.gov/std/treatment/2006/rr5511.pdf. [Accessed December, 2015].
5. Chapel TA. The signs and symptoms of secondary syphilis. Sex Transm Dis. 1980;7(4):161-4.
6. Chosidow O. Scabies and pediculosis. Lancet. 2000;355(9206):819-21.
7. Cobbold RJ, Macdonald A. Molluscum contagiosum as a sexually transmitted disease. Practitioner. 1970;204:416-9.
8. Cribier B, Frances C, Chosidow O. Treatment of lichen planus. An evidence-based medicine analysis of efficacy. Arch Dermatol. 1998;134(12):1521-30.
9. Criteria for diagnosis of Behcet's disease. International Study Group for Behcet's Disease. Lancet. 1990;335(8697):1078-80.
10. Curtin JP, Rubin SC, Jones WB, Hoskins WJ, Lewis JL Jr. Paget's disease of the vulva. Gynecol Oncol. 1990;39(3):374-7.
11. Dalziel KL, Millard PR, Wojnarowska F. The treatment of vulval lichen sclerosus with a very potent topical steroid (clobetasol propionate 0.05%) cream. Br J Dermatol. 1991;124(5):461-4.
12. de Chambrun MP, Wechsler B, Geri G, Cacoub P, Saadoun D. New insights into the pathogenesis of Behcet's disease. Autoimmun Rev. 2011;11(10):687-98.
13. de Villiers EM. Human papillomavirus. Introduction. Semin Cancer Biol. 1999;9(6):377.

14. Dubey S, Sharma R, Maheshwari V. Scrotal calcinosis: Idiopathic or dystrophic? Dermatol Online J. 2010;16(2):5.
15. Edwards L. Imiquimod in clinical practice. J Am Acad Dermatol. 2000;43(1 Pt 2):S12-7.
16. Fleischer AB Jr, Parrish CA, Glenn R, Feldman SR. Condylomata acuminata (genital warts): patient demographics and treating physicians. Sex Transm Dis. 2001;28(11):643-7.
17. Fraser CM, Norris SJ, Weinstock GM, White O, Sutton GG, Dodson R, et al. Complete genome sequence of Treponema pallidum, the syphilis spirochete. Science. 1998;281(5375):375-88.
18. Global prevalence and incidence of selected curable sexually transmitted infections overview and estimates. New York, USA: World Health Organization; 2001.
19. Guerry SL, Bauer HM, Klausner JD, Branagan B, Kerndt PR, Allen BG, et al. Recommendations for the selective use of herpes simplex virus type 2 serological tests. Clin Infect Dis. 2005;40(1):38-45.
20. Guidelines for the management of sexually transmitted infections. Geneva, Switzerland: World Health Organization; 2003.
21. Hook EW 3rd, Martin DH, Stephens J, Smith BS, Smith K. A randomized, comparative pilot study of azithromycin versus benzathine penicillin G for treatment of early syphilis. Sex Transm Dis. 2002;29(8):486-90.
22. Ingall D, Sánchez PJ. Syphilis. In: Remington JS, Klein JO (Eds). Infectious Diseases of the Fetus and Newborn Infant, 5th edition. Philadelphia: WB Saunders; 2001. pp. 643-81.
23. Jackson DJ, Rakwar JP, Bwayo JJ, Kreiss JK, Moses S. Urethral Trichomonas vaginalis infection and HIV-1 transmission. The Lancet. 1997;350(9084):1076.
24. James WD, Berger TG, Elston DM, Odom RB. Andrews' Diseases of the Skin: Clinical Dermatology, 10th edition. Philadelphia: Saunders Elsevier; 2006.
25. Jurstrand M, Christerson L, Klint M, Fredlund H, Unemo M, Herrmann B. Characterization of Chlamydia trachomatis by ompA sequencing and multilocus sequence typing (MLST) in a Swedish county before and after identification of the new variant. Sex Transm Infect. 2010;86:56-60.
26. Karthikeyan K. Treatment of scabies: newer perspectives. Postgrad Med J. 2005;81(951):7-11.
27. Katz DA, Berger JR, Duncan RC. Neurosyphilis: a comprehensive study of the effects of infection with human immunodeficiency virus. Arch Neurol. 1993;50:243-9.
28. Kingsley GH. Reactive arthritis: a paradigm for inflammatory arthritis. Clin Exp Rheumatol. 1993;11(8):S29-36.
29. Kumar B, Sharma R, Rajagopalan M, Radotra BD. Plasma cell balanitis: clinical and histopathological features—response to circumcision. Genitourin Med. 1995;71(1):32-4.
30. Lewis DA. Chancroid: clinical manifestations, diagnosis, and management. Sex Transm Infect. 2003;79(1):68-71.

Bibliography

31. Libois A, De Wit S, Poll B, Garcia F, Florence E, Del Rio A, et al. HIV and syphilis: when to perform a lumbar puncture. Sex Transm Dis. 2007;34(3): 141-4.
32. Lisboa C, Costa A, Ricardo E, Santos A, Azevedo F, Pina-Vaz C, et al. Genital candidosis in heterosexual couples. J Eur Acad Dermatol Venereol. 2010;25(2):145-51.
33. Mabey D, Ackers J, Adu-Sarkodie Y. Trichomonas vaginalis infection. Sex Transm Infect. 2006;82(Suppl 4):26-7.
34. Mabey D, Peeling RW. Lymphogranuloma venereum. Sex Transm Infect. 2002;78(2):90-2.
35. Marra CM. Deja vu all over again: when to perform a lumbar puncture in HIV-infected patients with syphilis. Sex Transm Dis. 2007;34(3):145-6.
36. Meffert JJ, David BM, Grinwood RD. Lichen sclerosus. J Am Acad Dermatol. 1995;32:393-416.
37. Melville J, Sniffen S, Crosby R, Salazar L, Whittington W, Dithmer-Schreck D, et al. Psychosocial impact of serological diagnosis of herpes simplex virus type 2: a qualitative assessment. Sex Transm Infect. 2003;79(4):280-5.
38. Moore RA, Edwards JE, Hopwood J, Hicks D. Imiquimod for the treatment of genital warts: a quantitative systematic review. BMC Infect Dis. 2001;1:3.
39. Morse SA. Etiology of genital ulcer disease and its relationship to HIV infection. Sex Transm Dis. 1999;26(1):63-5.
40. Musher DM, Hamill RJ, Baughn RE. Effect of human immunodeficiency virus (HIV) infection on the course of syphilis and on the response to treatment. Ann Intern Med. 1990;113(11):872-81.
41. Noer HR. An "experimental" epidemic of Reiter's syndrome. JAMA. 1996;198(7):693-8.
42. Nugent RP, Krohn MA, Hillier SL. Reliability of diagnosing bacterial vaginosis is improved by a standardized method of gram stain interpretation. J Clin Microbiol. 1991;29(2):297-301.
43. O'Farrell N. Donovanosis: an update. Int J STD AIDS. 2001;12(7):423-7.
44. Ohno S, Ohguchi M, Hirose S, Matsuda H, Wakisaka A, Aizawa M. Close association of HLA-Bw51 with Behcet's disease. Arch Ophthalmol. 1982;100(9):1455-8.
45. Paz-Bailey G, Ramaswamy M, Hawkes SJ, Geretti AM. Herpes simplex virus type 2: epidemiology and management options in developing countries. Sex Transm Infect. 2007;83(1):16-22.
46. Petrin D, Delgaty K, Bhatt R, Garber G. Clinical and microbiological aspects of Trichomonas vaginalis. Clin Microbiol Rev. 1998;11(2)300-17.
47. Phipps WSM, Saracino M, Magaret A, Selke S, Remington M, Huang ML, et al. Persistent genital herpes simplex virus-2 shedding years following the first clinical episode. J Infect Dis. 2011;203(2):180-7.
48. Powell FC, Bjornsson J, Doyle JA, Cooper AJ. Genital Paget's disease and urinary tract malignancy. J Am Acad Dermatol. 1985;13(1):84-90.
49. Richens J. Donovanosis (granuloma inguinale). Sex Transm Infect. 2006; 82(4):21-2.

50. Scheinfeld N, Lehman DS. An evidence-based review of medical and surgical treatments of genital warts. Dermatol Online J. 2006;12(3):5.
51. Schmid GP. Treatment of chancroid, 1997. Clin Infect Dis. 1999;28 Suppl 1:S14-20.
52. Shaw K, Puri K, Ruiz-Deya G, Hellstrom WJG. Racial consideration in the evaluation of Peyronie's disease. J Urol. 2001;165(170):687.
53. Smith GL, Bunker CB, Dinneen MD. Fournier's gangrene. BJU. 1998;81(3): 347-55.
54. Surendran KAK, Bhat RM, Boloor R, Nandakishore B, Sukumar D. A clinical and mycological study of dermatophytic infections. Indian J Dermatol. 2014;59(3):262-7.
55. Syed TS, Braverman PK. Vaginitis in adolescents. Adolesc Med Clin. 2004;15(2):235-51.
56. Tal R, Hall MS, Alex B, Choi J, Mulhall JP. Peyronie's disease in teenagers. J Sex Med. 2012;9(1):302-8.
57. Trees DL, Morse SA. Chancroid and Haemophilus ducreyi: an update. Clin Microbiol Rev. 1995;8(3):357-75.
58. Vohra S, Badlani G. Balanitis and balanoposthitis. Urol Clin North Am. 1992;19(1):143-7.
59. Wald A, Corey L, Cone R, Hobson A, Davis G, Zeh J. Frequent genital herpes simplex virus 2 shedding in immunocompetent women: effect of acyclovir treatment. J Clin Invest. 1997;99(5):1092-7.
60. Wiley DJ, Douglas J, Beutner K, Cox T, Fife K, Moscicki AB, et al. External genital warts: diagnosis, treatment, and prevention. Clin Infect Dis. 2002;35(Suppl 2):S210-24.
61. World Health Organization. Sexually transmitted diseases: Diagnostics initiative. [online] Available from: www.who.int/std_diagnostics.

Index

Page numbers followed by *f* refer to figure and *t* refer to table.

A

5-fluorouracil 67
   in Erythroplasia of Queyrat (EQ) 187
   side effects 68
Acetarsol pessaries
   in *Trichomonas vaginalis* 34
Acquired lymphangioma 204
Acrdermatitis enteropathica 182*f*
   with intertrigo 183*f*
Acyclovir
   in erythema multiforme 121
   in herpes genitalis in pregnancy 84
   in HSV infection 81
   in HSV-1 infection 80
   in neonatal herpes 85
Allergic contact dermatitis 166
   sources of 173*t*
   symptoms 167
Angiokeratomas 8, 9
Angiolymphoid hyperplasia 212*f*
Anogenital warts 59
Anthralin
   in psoriasis 166
Aphthous ulceration 146
Aqueous benzylpenicillin
   for congenital syphilis 49
   for neurosyphilis 49
Asaccharolytica 152
Atopic eczema 173
Atrophic vulvovaginitis 184
   treatment 185
Azathioprine
   in pemphigus 117
   in Reiter's syndrome 159
Azithromycin
   in chancroid 18
   in granuloma inguinale 22*t*

B

Bacterial vaginosis (BV) 26
   Amsel criteria 27
   Nugent score 28
   risk factors 26
   symptomatic 26
   treatment recommendations 28
Bacteroides ureolyticus 152
Balanitis 150
   aerobic infection 152
   allergic 154
   anaerobic infection 152
   candidal 150
   circinata 158, 159
   mycobacterial 153
   protozoal 153
   spirochetal 154
   syphilitic 154
   ulcerative 154
   viral infection 154
Balanoposthitis 150
   causes 151*t*
Bartholin's gland diseases 207
   treatment 208
Basal cell carcinoma (BCC) 195
Basement membrane zone (BMZ) 116
Behcet's disease 145
   aphthous ulceration 146
   clinical features 146
   differential diagnosis 148
   distiction from Reiter's syndrome 146
   erythema nodosum 148
   etiology 145
   joint manifestations 148
   ocular 147
   pathology 146
   pyoderma gangrenosum 149

treatment 150
Benign scrotal masses 209
Benzathine benzylpenicillin
   for syphilis 48, 49
Benzyl benzoate
   in scabies 16
Borrelia burgdorferi 34, 145
Bowenoid papulosis 187
   histopathology 188
Bowenoid papulosis (BP) 186
Bowen's disease 186
Bubo aspiration 95
   fluctuant bubo 95
   nonfluctuant bubo 95
Bullous dermatoses 7, 116
Buschke-Lowenstein tumor 53
BV *See* bacterial vaginosis (BV)

C

Calymmatobacterium granulomatis 19
   structure 19
Candida albicans 150
Candidal balanitis 101, 102*f*
   treatment 102
Candidal intertrigo 101
Capsaicin
   in ulvar vestibulitis syndrome 218
Carbon dioxide laser therapy
   in cervical cancer 67
Carcinoma cuniculatum 60
Cayenne pepper spots 156
Ceftriaxone
   in chancroid 18
      recommended regimens 18
   in granuloma inguinale 22*t*
Cephalexin
   erysipelas 109
Cervical cancer 59
   and human papillomavirus 59
   carbon dioxide laser therapy 67
   cryotherapy 65
   differential diagnosis 62
   electrosurgery 66
   surgical scissor excision 66
   treatment 62
Cervical cellular abnormalities 53
Cervical dysplasia 61
Chancroid 16

clinical features 16
diagnosis 17
   methods 17
extragenital cases of 17
treatment 18
Chlamydia trachomatis 22, 50, 96
   DNA amplification assays for 25
Chloramphenicol
   in granuloma inguinale 22*t*
Chronic idiopathic anal pain 217
Chronic inflammation of tunica albuginea (CITA) *See* Peyronie's disease
Chronic perianal pain 217
Cicatricial pemphigoid (CP) 119
   diagnosis 120
   direct immunofluorescence (DIF)
      findings 120
   erosions in 119
   genital involvement 119
      in men 119
      in women 119
   meatal stenosis 119
   phimosis in 119
   steroids in 120
   steroid sparing drugs 120
   treatment 120
Cidofovir
   in HSV-1 infection 81
Ciprofloxacin
   in chancroid 18
   in granuloma inguinale 22*t*
Clindamycin
   for bacterial vaginosis 28
CLM *See* cutaneous larva migrans (CLM)
Clotrimazole
   in candidal balanitis 102
   in vulvovaginal candidiasis 105
Coccygodynia descending perineum
   pain 217
Congenital melanocytic nevus I 209*f*
Coronal sulcus 2
Corticosteroids
   in pemphigus 117
   in Reiter's syndrome 159
Corynebacterium minutissimum 99
Corynebacterium tenuis 107
Cotrimoxazole
   in granuloma inguinale 22*t*
CP *See* cicatricial pemphigoid (CP)

Index

Crohn's disease 141
Cryotherapy
   in cervical cancer 65
   side effects 65
Cutaneous larva migrans (CLM) 113
   treatment 113
Cutaneous lymphangiectasia 204
Cyclic vulvovaginitis 215
   symptoms 215
Cyclophosphamide
   in pemphigus 117
Cyproterone acetate
   in hidradenitis suppurativa (HS) 144

D

Dapsone
   in linear immunoglobulin A
     dermatosis (LAD) 127
Dark-field microscopy 89
   method of specimen collection for 89
DB *See* donovan bodies (DB)
Diaper dermatitis 169f, 175
   clinical finding 175
   treatment 175
Diaper rash *See* diaper dermatitis
Dicloxacillin
   erysipelas 109
Donovan bodies (DB) 19
Donovanosis *See* granuloma inguinale
   (donovanosis)
Dowling-Degos disease 141
Doxycycline
   for syphilis 48, 49
   in granuloma inguinale 22t
   lymphogranuloma venereum 25

E

EBA *See* epidermolysis bullosa acquisita
   (EBA)
Econazole
   in candidal balanitis 102
   in vulvovaginal candidiasis 105
Ectopic sebaceous glands 8
Ecurrent respiratory papillomatosis 52
Eczema 166
E genes 52
Electrosurgery
   in cervical cancer 66

Elephantiasis 20
EMPD *See* extramammary Paget's
   disease
Endometriosis 209
Entamoeba histolytica 153
Enterobius vermicularis 106
Epidermolysis bullosa acquisita
   (EBA) 127
   clinical features 128
   diagnosis 128
   treatment 129
Erysipelas 109
   lesions 109
   treatment 109
Erythema multiforme (EM) 120
   HSV coinfection 121
   iris lesions 121
   lesions in 121
   treatment 121
Erythema nodosum
   in Behcet's disease 148
Erythrasma 99
   treatment 100
   with candidal intertrigo 101f
Erythromycin
   erysipelas 109
   in chancroid 18
   in erythrasma 100
   in granuloma inguinale 22t
   in lymphogranuloma venereum 25
   in syphilis 48
Erythroplasia of Queyrat (EQ) 186
   differential diagnoses 186
   histopathology 187
Escherichia coli 106
Ethinylestradiol
   in hidradenitis suppurativa (HS) 144
Etretinate
   in Reiter's syndrome 159
Extramammary Paget's disease 189
   histopathological findings 189
   perianal 189
   vulval 189

F

Famciclovir
   in HSV infection 81
   in HSV-1 infection 80

Genital Dermatoses

Familial benign chronic pemphigus *See* Hailey-Hailey disease
FDE *See* fixed drug eruption (FDE)
FG *See* Fournier's gangrene (FG)
Fibroepithelial polyp 209
Finasteride
   in hidradenitis suppurativa (HS) 144
Fixed drug eruption (FDE) 122
   common sites 123
   histopathological differentiation 125
   treatment 125
Flucloxacillin
   linear immunoglobulin a dermatosis (LAD) 127
Fluconazole
   in candidal balanitis 102
   in vulvovaginal candidiasis 105
Fluorescent treponemal antibody absorption double staining tests 45
Fluorescent treponemal antibody absorption test 45
Folliculitis 107
   lesions in 107
Fordyce spots 8
Fournier's gangrene (FG) 202
   causes 203
   suppurative bacterial infection 203
Furazolidone
   in *Trichomonas vaginalis* 34
Furunculosis 107
Fusidic acid
   in erythrasma 100
Fusobacterium spp 152

G

Gardnerella vaginalis 26, 103, 152
Gartner's duct cyst 209
Genital HPV infection 53
   clinical manifestations of 53
   risk factors 53
Genitalia
   female 2
      anatomical variants 8
      anatomy of 4*f*
      clinical examination 6
   male 2
      anatomical variants 8
      anatomy 3*f*
      clinical examination 6

Genital pain syndrome 7, 214
Genital ulcer disease (GUD) 50
Genital ulcer disease-herpetic (GUD-H) 51
Genital ulcer disease- non herpetic (GUD-NH) 51
Genital wart 50
   morphologic types 53
      condylomata acuminata 54
      flat papules 53
      giant condyloma 53
      keratotic warts 53
      smooth papules 53
   sites 59
   symptoms 59
Genital warts 53
   in pregnancy 68
Giant condyloma of Buschke and Lowenstein 60
Giemsa stain 93
   donovanosis 93
   genital herpes 93
   molluscum contagiosum 94
Gonorrhea 90
   method of sample collection 91
      endocervical swab 91
      pharyngeal swab 92
      rectal swab 92
      urethral swab 91, 92
      vaginal swab 92
Gram staining 90
   bacterial vaginosis 93
   gonorrhea 90
Granuloma inguinale (donovanosis) 19
   clinical features 20
   diagnosis 21
      Giemsa stain 21
      Leishman stain 21
      polymerase chain reaction techniques 21
   drugs used 22*t*
   lesions 20
      cicatricial 20
      hypertrophic or verrucous 20
      locations 20
      nodular 20
      ulcerovegetative 20
   treatment 21
Groove sign 23

Index

H

Haemophilus ducreyi 16, 96
Haemophilus influenzae 106
Hailey-hailey disease 118
    biopsy in 118
    diagnosis 118
    lesions in 118
    precipitating factors 118
    treatment 118
Helicase-primase inhibitors 87
Helicobacter pylori 145
Hemangiopericytoma 209
Henderson-Patterson inclusion bodies 12
Herpes genitalis 70
    clinical features 72
    counseling 86
    differential diagnosis 77
    drug resistance 85
    in pregnancy 84
    investigations 77
    pathophysiology 71
    prevention 86
    primary 72
        symptoms 72
    recurrences 75
    treatment 79
        for first episode 81
        for recurrence 81
        of severe disease 83
    vaccines 87
    with secondary infection 73, 76f
Herpes gestationis *See* pemphigoid gestationis
Herpes simplex 154
Herpes simplex virus (HSV) 70
    direct fluorescent antibody test (DFA) 78
    first episode 71
    nonprimary infection 71
    polymerase chain reaction 78
    primary infection 71
    rapid assay 78
    recurrence 71
    resistance
        acyclovir-resistant strains 85
    serologic assays 79
    serology 79
    transmission 71
    type 1 70
    type 2 70
    viral culture 77
Hidradenitis suppurativa (HS) 141
    clinical features 142
    complications 144
    Crohn's disease 141
    differential diagnosis 144
    dowling-degos disease 141
    etiology 141
    severity of 142
    treatment 144
HPV *See* Human papillomavirus
HPV 18 60
HS *See* hidradenitis suppurativa (HS)
HSV 96 *See* Herpes simplexvirus
Human papillomavirus 16, 18, 52, 59, 60, 154
    diagnosis 61
    human immunodeficiency virus coinfection 83
    untreated
        complications of 60
Human papillomavirus vaccines 68
    bivalent vaccine (HPV2) 68
    quadrivalent vaccine (HPV4) 68

I

Imidazole
    in candidal balanitis 102
Imiquimod
    in cervical cancer 63
    in erythroplasia of queyrat (EQ) 187
    mechanism of action 63
    treated patients 63
Immunofluorescence
    method of specimen collection for 95
Immunofluorescence staining 77
Immunomodulatory drug
    in pemphigus 117
Incontenentia pigmenti 212f
Infantile haemangioma 211f
Infantile intertrigo 183
Inflammatory conditions 7
Interferon 2β
    in Peyronie's disease 200

Genital Dermatoses

Intertrigo
   acrodermatitis enteropathica 183f
   causes 181
   infantile 183
Intra-anal warts 59
Intraepithelial neoplasia 186, 188f
Irritant contact dermatitis 171, 168f, 171f
Itraconazole
   in vulvovaginal candidiasis 105
Ivermectin
   in scabies 16
   mode of action 16

J

Jock itch 97

K

Kaposi varicelliform eruption 115f
Keratoderma blennorrhagicum 158
Klebsiella granulomatis 21
Koebner's phenomenon 139f
KOH mount 94
   bacterial vaginosis 94
   genital candidiasis 94
KOH wet mount-whiff test
   in bacterial vaginosis 27

L

Labia majora 3
LAD *See* linear immunoglobulin a dermatosis (LAD)
Leiomyoma 209
Leprosy 153
Leptospira 34
Leptospirosis 34
LGV *See* lymphogranuloma venereum (LGV)
Lichen planus 137
   clinical features 138
   histopathology 140
   treatment 141
   types of 138
Lichen sclerosus et atrophicus (LSA) 131, 133, 135f
   characteristic sites 132
   circumcision in 137
   clinical features 132
   differential diagnosis 137
   etiology 131
   histopathology 136
   keyhole or hourglass appearance 132
   orthohyperkeratosis in 136
   perianal lesions 132
   prognosis 136
   treatment 137
   vitiligo with 134f
Lichen simplex 173
Lindane
   in scabies 16
Linear immunoglobulin A dermatosis (LAD) 126
   clinical features 126
   diagnosis 126
   lesions in 126
   treatment 127
Localised epidermal nevus 210f
Lozenge keratinocytes 156
LSA *See* lichen sclerosus et atrophicus (LSA)
Lupus vulgaris (LV) 111
   lesions in 111
   of gluteal skin 112f
Lyme disease 34
Lymphangiectasia 205f
Lymphangioma circumscriptum (LC) 206
Lymphogranuloma venereum (LGV) 22
   anorectal involvement 23
   clinical course of 23
   clinical features 23
   diagnosis 24
   differential diagnosis 24
   inguinal form 23
   primary stage 23
   proctitis 23
   secondary stage 23
   tertiary stage 24
   treatment 25

M

Malakoplakia 108
   cutaneous 108
Malassezia 174
Malathion
   in pediculosis pubis 13
Malignant diseases of genitalia 7
Malignant melanoma 197
Mammary Paget's disease (PD) 189

Index

MC *See* molluscum contagiosum (MC)
Methotrexate
   in pemphigus 117
   in Reiter's syndrome 159
Metronidazole 28
   for bacterial vaginosis 28
   safety in pregnany 33
Metronidazole
   in trichomonas vaginalis 32
Michaelis-gutmann bodies 108
Miconazole
   in candidal balanitis 102
   in vulvovaginal candidiasis 105
Microimmunofluorescence (MIF) test 25
Molluscum contagiosum (MC) 10, 11*f*
   diagnosis 12
   differential diagnosis 11
   lesion 10
   spread 10
   treatment 12
Molluscum contagiosum virus (MCV) 10
   types 10
Multiple scrotal cyst 201*f*
Mycobacterium smegmatis 155
Mycophenolate mofetil in
      pemphigus 117
Mycoplasma genitalium 50

N

Neonatal herpes 85
Neurofibromas 209
Neurofibromatosis 211
Neurosyphilis 36, 38
   early 39
   late 39
   symptomatic 40
N. Gonorrhoeae 96
Nikolsky's sign 122
Nitroimidazole
   in *Trichomonas vaginalis* 32
Nitroimidazoles
   for bacterial vaginosis 28
Nongonococcal urethritis 92
Nonsyphilitic spirochetes 154
Nontreponemal test 39
Norfloxacin
   in granuloma inguinale 22*t*
Norwegian scabies 14
Nugent score 28

O

Oligoarthritis 158
Oral florid papillomatosis 60

P

Papanicolaou-stained smear
      technique 28
Pap test 61
Paramesonephric duct cyst 209
Paromomycin
   in *Trichomonas vaginalis* 34
Partial penectomy 201
Pediculosis pubis 12
   diagnosis 13
   management 13
   spread 13
Pemphigoid gestationis 129
Pemphigus 116
   cause 117
   chronic 117
   complications 117
   immunomodulatory drug in 117
   treatment 117
Pemphigus foliaceus 116
Pemphigus vulgaris 116
   lesions in 117
Penciclovir
   in HSV-1 infection 80
Penile genital wart 56*f*
Penile horn 200
   etiology 200
   partial penectomy 201
   treatment 201
Penile intraepithelial neoplasia (PIN) 186
Penile papules 8
Penile warts 59
Penilodynia 216
Penis 2
Peptostreptococcus 144
Perianal abscess 110
   cardinal signs of inflammation 110
   treatment 110
Perianal syndrome 217
Perianal warts 55*f*, 59
Permethrin
   in pediculosis pubis 13
   in scabies 16
Peyronie's disease 198

Genital Dermatoses

abnormal curvature of penis 199f
pathogenesis 198
vacuum therapy 200
PG See pemphigoid gestationis
Phthirus pubis 12
 transmission 12
Pidermophyton floccosum 97
Pimecrolimus
 in lichen sclerosus et atrophicus (LSA) 137
 in psoriasis 166
Pityriasis versicolor 99
PKMB See pseudoepitheliomatous, keratotic, and micaceous balanitis (PKMB)
Plasma cell balanitis 155
Podophyllin 64
Podophyllotoxin
 in cervical cancer 62
Podophyllum emodi 64
Podophyllum peltatum 64
Polymerase chain reaction
 methods for 96
Prednisone
 in erythema multiforme 121
Premalignant dermatoses 7
Procaine benzylpenicillin
 for neurosyphilis 49
 for syphilis 48, 49
Proctalgia fugax 217
Propionibacterium acnes 144
Prozone reactions 43
Pseudoepitheliomatous, keratotic, and micaceous balanitis (PKMB) 190
 pathogenesis of 190
 treatment 191
Psoriasis 160
 clinical features 160
 dry scaly plaque of 160f
 flexural 161f
 genital 162, 162f
 involving groin 164f
 lesions 160
 perianal area 164f
 treatment 165
 vulvar 160
Pyoderma gangrenosum (PG) 149, 149f

R

Rapid plasma reagin (RPR) 43, 44
Rapid tests 46
Reiter's syndrome 146, 157
 balanitis circinata 158
 etiology 158
 keratoderma blennorrhagicum 158
 laboratory findings 159
 mucocutaneous involvement 158
 oligoarthritis 158
 oral involvement 159
 pathogenesis 158
 treatment 159
 ultraviolet B (UVB) phototherapy 159

S

Sarcoptes scabiei 13
Scabies 13
 clinical features 14
 diagnosis 15
 human immunodeficiency virus (HIV) infection 14
 incubation period 14
 route of transmission 14
 topical treatments 16
 treatment 16
 with secondary infection 15f
Scrofuloderma 111
 clinical features 111
Scrotal calcinosis (SC) 201
 calcification of epidermal cysts 202
 calcification of Dartos muscle 202
 pathogenesis 202
 recurrence 202
Scrotal eczema 168
Scrotodynia 216
Sebaceous gland
 hyperplasia 9
Seborrheic dermatitis 174
Seborrheic eczema 174
 cutaneous manifestation 174
 diagnosis 174
 symptoms 174
Sexually transmitted infections
 methods of specimen collection 88
Sexually transmitted infections (STIs) 5
Sinecatechins 15% ointment
 in cervical cancer 64

Index

SJS *See* Stevens-Johnson syndrome (SJS)
SJS-TEN overlap 122
Southern blot hybridization technique 61
Squamous cell carcinoma (SCC) 60, 192
   clinical features 193
   histology 193
   penile 193*f*
      TNM classification 194
      treatment 195
   total penectomy 195
Squamous cell hyperplasia 175, 176*f*
   lichen sclerosus 177*f*
   with secondary changes 178*f*
Staphyloccocus aureus 153
Stevens-Johnson syndrome (SJS) 121, 122, 123*f*
   symptoms 122
   treatment 122
STIs *See* sexually transmitted infections
Streptococci 153
Streptomycin
   in granuloma inguinale 22
Sulfamethoxypyridazine
   in linear immunoglobulin A dermatosis (LAD) 127
Sulfasalazine
   in Reiter's syndrome 159
Surgical scissor excision
   in cervical cancer 66
Syndrome of esthiomene 24
Syphilis 34
   acquired 34
   and pregnancy 39
   asymptomatic 39
   cardiovascular 38
   chancre 36
   congenital 34
      clinical manifestations 40
   congenital 36
   early latent 35
   gummatous 38
   human immunodeficiency virus 40
   incubating 35
   late latent 35
   latent 37
   neurosyphilis 36
   primary 35
   secondary 35, 37
   tertiary 38
   treatment 48
   uncommon 38
Syphilitic balanitis 154

T

Tacrolimus
   in lichen sclerosus et atrophicus (LSA) 137
Taphylococcus aureus 107, 109
Tazarotene
   in psoriasis 166
TB colliquativa cutis 111
TEN *See* toxic epidermal necrolysis (TEN)
Tetracycline
   in erythrasma 100
   in granuloma inguinale 22*t*
   in lymphogranuloma venereum 25
   in syphilis 48, 49
Tinea cruris 97
   clinical features 98
   diagnosis 98
   differential diagnosis 99
   etiology 97
   KOH wet mount 98
   treatment 99
Tinidazole
   for bacterial vaginosis 28
   in trichomonas vaginalis 32
Tissue inhibitors of metalloproteinases (TIMPs) 199
TNM classification
   of squamous cell carcinoma, penile 194
Toluidine red unheated serum test (TRUST) 43, 44
Total penectomy 195
Toxic epidermal necrolysis (TEN) 121, 122
   Nikolsky's sign 124*f*
   symptoms 122
Transport media for culture 96
Treponemal serological tests 44
Treponema pallidum 34
   dark-field microscopy 42
   diagnosis 41
   direct fluorescent antibody test for 42

nontreponemal serological tests 43
nucleic acid amplification method 43
Treponema pallidum particle
    agglutination test 45
Trichloroacetic acid (TCA) 64
    side effects of 64
Trichomonas 153
Trichomonas vaginalis (TV) 28, 96, 103
    diagnosis 30
        females 30
        males 31
    infection symptoms 29
    laboratory investigations 31
        culture 31
        microscopy 31
        molecular detection 31
    management 32
    spread 29
    structure of 29f
    treatment 32
Trichomoniasis 28
Trichomycosis pubis 107
    treatment 107
Trichophyton mentagrophytes 97
Trichophyton rubrum 97
Trichophyton verrucosum 97
Tuberculosis 111
    verrucosa cutis 111
Tzanck smear 77

U

Ultraviolet B (UVB) phototherapy
    in Reiter's syndrome 159
Unheated serum reagin (USR) test 43
Urogenital triangle 2

V

Vagina
    benign neoplasms 208
Valacyclovir
    in herpes genitalis in pregnancy 84
Valacyclovir
    in HSV-1 infection 80

in HSV associated HIV infection 83
in HSV infection 81
Vancomycin
    in linear immunoglobulin A
        dermatosis (LAD) 126
Varicella 115f
Venereal disease research laboratory 44
Verrucous carcinoma (VC) 60
Vestibular glands 4
Vestibular papillae 8
Vitamin D analogues
    in psoriasis 166
Vitiligo 178
    with leucotrichia 179f
    with LSA 180f
Vulvar intraepithelial neoplasia (VIN) 188
Vulvar vestibulitis syndrome 215
    cause 216
    clinical findings 216
    treatment 217
Vulvar warts 59
Vulvodynia 214
Vulvovaginal candidiasis (VVC) 102
    clinical features 103
    treatment 104
Vulvovaginitis 102
VVC *See* vulvovaginal
    candidiasis (VVC)

W

Western blot 46
Wet mount 94

Z

Zoon's balanitis 155
    cayenne pepper spots 156
    circumcision 157
    clinical features 156
    diagnosis 156
    differential diagnosis 157
    etiology 155
    pathology 156
    treatment 157